AMBULANCE!

AMBULANCE!

Glen McCoy

David & Charles
Newton Abbot   London   North Pomfret (Vt)

British Library Cataloguing in Publication Data

McCoy, Glen
  Ambulance!
  1. London—Ambulance Service
  I. Title
  362.1'8'09421   RA996.G/

  ISBN 0–7153–8182–2

Filmset in Monophoto Plantin
by Latimer Trend & Company Ltd, Plymouth
and printed in Great Britain
by Redwood Burn, Trowbridge, Wiltshire
for David & Charles (Publishers) Limited
Brunel House Newton Abbot Devon

Published in the United States of America
by David & Charles Inc
North Pomfret Vermont 05053 USA

Contents

*To the professional Ambulancemen and Women of
Great Britain*

Foreword

Dirty, dangerous and unappreciated: that might be an apt description of ambulance-service work. Nevertheless, the ambulanceman must handle every call efficiently and treat every case as a special one. I have had the pleasure of knowing the author of this book for some years since he entered the Ambulance Service. He was trained at the same time as my eldest son, and I have watched them both develop into caring and considerate adults. I feel that part of the reason for this is the work they do in emergency services.

Those who frequently pass an ambulance on its way to an emergency, its lights flashing and siren going, rarely pause to think of the implications or provisions such a service requires. It is, as in many things, only when we require help that we even consider what it must be like to deal with bad road accidents, drunks or dangerously distraught and disturbed patients. The modern ambulanceman, however, deals with many such cases in his normal working day, particularly if the work is in a large city.

In one particular case I know of, an ambulance crew was called to deal with a violent patient accused of wounding another in a squat; ambulancemen were faced with an armed attacker and a badly bleeding patient. Only their calm approach prevented a bad case of wounding developing into a mass assault. They are needed to deal with appalling accidents involving children. The infant whose baby-bouncer collapses, driving a steel rivet into its tiny form, is in desperate need of urgent aid as it is transported to the hospital. On a happier note, most ambulances have also produced their fair share of newborn babies in transit.

Modern emergency methods often mean that a patient

must be kept alive either by resuscitation or medication until being handed over to an accident and emergency unit. The skills needed by the ambulance crew are, therefore, of a very high standard indeed and differ from day to day. In fact, since my youth, ambulance work has changed radically, from the rather routine task of conveying patients to hospital to the much tougher, occasionally dangerous, ambulance job of the 1980s. The modern ambulanceman is at the sharp end, and it is not always realized that he is a trained operative capable of giving life-support that can make the difference between life and death. Yet ambulance services are still not regarded by the general public in the same light as the Police and Fire Brigade, often the only 999 services considered as important. The Ambulance Service is often remembered or appreciated only by those in acute medical emergencies.

Glen McCoy has set out to rectify this situation, attempting to provide precisely the sort of information that is vital for the general public. Speaking as I do in the House of Commons on health matters, and watching day-to-day as an ambulanceman's Mum the working of the Service, I increasingly appreciate the men and women who do this vital job. What Glen has set out to achieve has never been produced in this way before. If it succeeds in bringing home to the general public exactly what his job and the job of many of his fellow workers is all about, then I think he will have performed a signal service to us all.

Gwyneth Dunwoody, MP
House of Commons

Introduction

If I were to tell someone that I had a milk round, repaired television sets, sold encyclopaedias or flew 747 aircraft, they would immediately conjure up a mental picture of my work. Nine times out of ten the image would be accurate, and no further explanation would be required. Yet this is rarely the case when I say 'I'm an ambulanceman'. Some enquire what exactly that involves, while others betray a lack of understanding or complete ignorance.

The only individuals who really appreciate what an ambulanceman's job entails are other ambulancemen and women. Even the people we work with closely, such as doctors, nurses, police officers and firemen, do not fully understand the nature of our work, the extent of the equipment we are trained to use or the level of medical know-how necessary in accident and emergency care.

Out on the battlefield of major incident or at the scene of a serious accident, ambulance personnel have to contend with any situation that faces them. There is no one to offer advice or make a difficult decision on their behalf. Sometimes they have to identify and locate a problem, then devise a solution. Such problems may occur in the street, on a roof-top, on a railway line or even underground. There is no sterile hospital environment for any medical treatment until the patient is safely within the ambulance. A crew will have to deal with whatever is pointed in its direction with the same efficiency, enthusiasm and calm. An aged tramp must be given as much sympathy and consideration as a young child; colour, creed, religion and politics are irrelevant.

Many may look upon me as a glorified taxi-driver, others as a surrogate doctor. But whatever my status, I am usually all there is between a medical crisis and hospital care. The treatment given at the scene of a call and subsequently in the ambulance often has a substantial effect on the patient's eventual recovery; without it he might not even survive long enough to reach hospital. This is particularly true for people with spinal injuries and serious coronary attacks, the badly injured victims of road accidents and patients who need immediate resuscitation measures.

The variety of cases ambulance personnel have to deal with is unlimited, and may range from cut fingers to decapitations. Training, as a result, has to be thorough and far exceeds the basic rudiments of first aid. These days professional ambulance staff are skilled technicians who specialise in emergency patient care. They form a vital link in a medical chain that is essential to any patient, promoting recovery where possible and sustaining basic life functions.

I hope the real work of ambulancemen and women, such a vital and integral part of our society, will become clearer on the pages that follow. The job is portrayed through real-life incidents and actual case histories.

I

Breaking Point

26 July 1979: 15.18 hours   Surging downwards, the solid 3-tonne mass smashed a path on to its unsuspecting victim below. The deafening thud set up vibrations throughout the factory warehouse, dying out gradually into an unnatural calm.

The split-second warning that had been bellowed to the young man beneath had undoubtedly saved his life; but now he lay trapped from the waist, pinned against a series of metal pipes that ran 6 feet above ground. The youth had been painting the pipe lines that now spanned the back of his body, which refused to submit to the pressure from above. The initial painful blow had given way to a general numb feeling below his thighs and a build-up of abdominal tenderness. Grimacing uncomfortably, he could hear an incessant sound of chattering voices that made little sense. As the noises became more erratic, echoing about him, he tried to adjust his blurred vision through watery eyes.

Workers in a state of near-panic rallied around the nineteen-year-old as chains were brought to bear upon the dense mass. Logic and reason seemed to elude the works team until someone eventually cried out above the cacophony of voices, 'For God's sake, someone call an ambulance!' Before professional assistance could be summoned, the unskilled rescue attempt failed miserably. During the effort to raise the heavy structure, a chain that was fastened loosely to the block slipped, allowing the metal mass to ram itself squarely upon the patient for a second time.

By now three magic numbers had been conjured from the office telephone: 999. As with all emergency calls made in the Greater London area, the operator connected it to the Central

Ambulance Control Centre at Waterloo, south London. Duty Control staff dealt with the ambulance request alongside the scores of other accident calls from all over the London area. This incident had occurred in Hayes, Middlesex, but all local ambulances were committed to other work at that time. The nearest ambulance available was situated at Hanwell, W7. At 15.26 the leading ambulanceman at Hanwell answered the direct emergency line. He took down the details of the accident on an official call sheet. 'Laboratory Warehouses, Bullsbridge Road, Hayes. Man trapped. Serious.'

The only 999 crew able to respond to this call was technically off duty at 15.00 hours and was waiting to be relieved by another oncoming shift. Nevertheless the crew was given the job and responded without delay. Steve Manhire and Dave Rees had been crewed together for some time now, and worked well as a team. Today Steve was medical attendant while Dave was in the driving seat. Both were in their twenties, and they had several years of experience between them.

Dave punched the ambulance out of the station smartly into the afternoon traffic along Boston Road. With blue beacons revolving and headlights dipped, the white vehicle wove through the lines of cars along the Uxbridge Road, its two-tone horns used when necessary to alert traffic ahead; most motorists helpfully made a path. On route, Red Base Ambulance Control radioed through to Hanwell 2, confirming details and stressing the severity of the accident. Dave's chest bit against his seat-belt as he leaned forward a little and increased the ambulance's speed, within safety limits. Wailing a route through Southall Broadway, the crew made towards the Coldharbour Lane intersection. As they approached the address they had been given, Dave noticed two men in overalls, waving frantically at them. The men pointed to the way into the warehouse complex, and Steve grabbed his immediate-aid kit, making ready to locate his patient. As Hanwell 2 drew up, Steve was beckoned inside a giant enclosure housing a myriad of pipes and stop-valves. Alighting from the cab, he briskly entered the building.

Sombre faces surrounded him and he could have sliced the stricken atmosphere with a knife as he moved to the site of the accident. Peering ahead, he was soon able to discern the shape of the young man extended uncomfortably upon the network of pipelines several feet above. Inches above his body hung a gigantic weight supported by a single chain.

Steve gritted his teeth: 'Shit,' he gasped under his breath, keeping hold of the calm professional behaviour instilled in him. Coming nearer, he could make out the victim's face. Leaving his satchel at ground level, he climbed up on the metal pipes stretched underneath the injured body. It was now possible to ascertain the extent of the visible injuries. The unfortunate lad looked like a piece of blancmange, with his right wrist tucked awkwardly behind him. His back was arched, and his lower limbs splayed in a deformed pattern. The right leg, which Steve realised was fractured, bore a nasty open wound.

The first communication with the patient came as eye-to-eye contact. The ambulanceman looked directly in his face, trying to show only reassurance in his own. Placing his hand gently on the boy's shoulder, Steve spoke softly. 'We're going to get you out of this mess—but you must trust us. What's your name?'

The patient responded with 'Noel' in between gasps for more air.

'OK, Noel, I'm Steve. Now tell me where it's hurting the most.' Noel managed to indicate that his back was extremely painful and that his abdomen ached. Steve's priorities soon became apparent. First he must support the patient's spine, and carefully he slid his left hand under the arched back. Pushing his hand right through, his own forearm became wedged and soon immovable, but he observed that this measure alleviated some of Noel's pain. Steve continued to evaluate the situation. 'Can you move your legs?'

The young patient, in a weak, shaky tone, drew Steve's attention to his abdomen. Using his other hand, Steve checked pulse, respiration and areas of tenderness, making a mental note of possible internal haemorrhage. Noel's pulse and respiration rate were high, and Steve's experience led him to suspect a ruptured spleen.

By now Dave had parked the ambulance in a convenient spot and had made his way through the small collection of workers. As he met his partner's gaze he could tell that the case was serious, even before he had set eyes on the patient. A plan of action was quickly worked out and set in motion. The crew was going to have to work hard if the lad's life was to be saved, as the internal bleeding, which became more evident with each passing minute, became a factor of great concern. Dave darted away to the ambulance, asking someone to clear the warehouse of onlookers. Grabbing the radio microphone, he called through on a priority basis, taking precedence over other mobiles on the busy airband.

'Go ahead, priority vehicle.'

'Roger. Hanwell 2, your 26 call. Request paramedic ambulance crew urgently and/or medical team. Also alert Fire Brigade. Patient trapped, and we may need heavy lifting gear.' There was a pause. 'Message received Hanwell 2. Police are also on their way. Red Base out.' It was 15.38, and on the tarmac outside Hillingdon Hospital Casualty Department an emergency ambulance—call sign Hillingdon 1—was 'green' and available. Having heard the last transmission it offered its services to transport a medical team. Control agreed. Meanwhile, at Greenford Ambulance Station, the emergency 'hot line' was being answered. Red Base ascertained that a paramedic crew was available and despatched Greenford 1 India to the scene (the suffix signified the crew had advanced training).

Back at the incident Dave had brought out the apparatus required to sustain their patient's life, but they urgently required a running intravenous drip, which only a paramedic ambulance crew or doctor could provide. It was critical that the casualty's condition was stabilised before he was moved, yet it was going to be a skilled four-man operation to remove him.

Entonox, a pain-relief gas, was soon set up for administration, and the boy took in deep breaths through a black face-mask connected to a small blue cylinder; the gas alleviated some of the pain that wracked the body trapped in the metal prison. Steve continually talked to his patient while he gripped the face-mask about his jaws; he knew the tension and stress the youth was experiencing, as through his cupped hands he could feel the uncontrolled vibrations of pain and fear tremble through to his own uneasy body. Noel's tightly shut eyes bore the weepy remains excreted from tear ducts.

After a few more minutes of entonox therapy, the ambulanceman decided that the strain of inhaling the static gas was becoming too much for the lad, and he asked his partner to organise a supply of free-flowing oxygen. Carefully withdrawing the entonox face-piece, Steve rechecked the pulse and respiration rate. Noel's colour was still far from normal.

The ambulance crew remained oblivious to the risk it was taking. Any movement or pressure exerted on that precariously suspended block would bring the 3-tonne mass crashing down for a third time, consuming perhaps three lives instead of one.

Dave extracted from a sterile packet a new green oxygen mask, connected to a portable oxygen pack. He passed it to his partner who gently eased the mask over Noel's drained expressionless face, using his right hand. His other hand and forearm felt crushed; he could sense 'pins and needles' at his finger tips, coupled with a slow, numbing feeling encompassing his entire limb. Despite this, his mind continually worked on a solution to the problem: how, when the time came, to get his patient out of this predicament.

The Fire Brigade sent out a rescue tender from Heston at 15.44. The Senior Fire Officer agreed with the ambulance crew not to touch the suspended block until the patient had received the necessary treatment, but the Officer offered to support it in the meantime, and Steve nodded agreement. The fire team set to work to move the specialised equipment into place while the ambulance crew worried about other matters. Steve was getting to know his patient well now, and the superficial level of the whispered conversation had altered; Noel began to respond to his chief rescuer like an old friend and talked about his family, girlfriend and future plans. But Steve observed the growing danger with each slipping second. The youth's condition was deteriorating, decreasing his chances of survival: something had to be done very soon to restore lost blood. Steve tried to summon every last conceivable word of optimism and reassurance without sounding as if he was muttering a string of clichés.

It was a six-minute journey for Greenford 1 India, which pulled up sharply on the gravel pathway alongside Hanwell 2. Just behind them came the medical team on the Hillingdon ambulance. Clive Swain, the Greenford attendant, radioed through to Red Base Control to state the position. He and his partner were subsequently instructed to return, since they were surplus to requirements now that the medical team was on scene. As Greenford slowly made its way out of the factory grounds, unaware of what was going on, the medical team gathered the essential apparatus. Led by ambulancemen James and Nugent, the doctor, nurse and theatre technician brought in their assortment of boxes and medical supplies. The casualty doctor, who was also a surgeon, a little bewildered away from the environment of a hospital, efficiently organised the delicate task ahead.

The tourniquet-like grip around Steve Manhire's arm tightened, but he tried not to think about his own discomfort. It seemed irrelevant in comparison with the problems his patient faced.

As the doctor edged as close to the gigantic block as he dared, Steve whispered a full report of the patient's present condition, with an assessment of possible injuries. The surgeon made his own diagnosis and, squinting at the sweating ambulanceman, signalled agreement with him. The nurse recorded the details: open fracture right tibia, fractured right wrist for possible amputation, fracture and dislocation at twelfth thoracic vertebra, paralysis of lower limbs, acute abdominal distress with probable ruptured spleen.

A tall limping man appeared from the small crowd that continued to stand outside the warehouse, brushing past the sea of shoulders until he could see the incident. A voice shouted at the groups of blue ambulance shirts around the metal block: 'It's the boy's father.' Steve winced at this and Dave, noticing his partner's reaction, turned to intercept the man. Throwing an arm about him, he said, 'There's nothing you can do; let's get him out first.' The man showed surprising calm in the circumstances and called out: 'How are you doing, Noel?' The youth feebly replied that he was all right. With that Dave insisted that the father should wait elsewhere and led him away to the sympathetic hands of his workmates.

The Hillingdon surgeon, Mr Phillips, had given Noel an injection of morphine sulphate, and Steve almost felt that he had been given the pain relief himself as he observed a wave of relief relax the boy's features. The therapy continued with an intravenous drip to replace the lost body fluid, and a blood sample was taken for urgent analysis. The police took the sample for cross-matching at the casualty unit and returned with two bags of the appropriate blood. Mr Phillips asked for a further four bags to be kept ready for use on arrival at hospital.

The next stage of the operation, raising the huge threatening mass, was going to be difficult and dangerous. But it was only when the Fire Brigade began to use the hoist that Steve really appreciated the gravity of the situation and his own part in it. As the weight was lifted inch by inch, he observed the medical staff and his own colleagues retire a few paces, but he could not take evasive action for his own safety. He and his patient had become one entity, bound under the object that was responsible for the accident. If it were to slip once more as it had done already, the incident would be permanently closed with the loss of two lives. Steve glanced above his head once and that proved too much. His back tingled and his blood ran cold. For the sake of his patient and of himself he had to concentrate on other matters. He smiled tentatively at the lad who was but a few years younger than himself, and Noel managed a faint grin of appreciation.

The cranking sound directly above the solid structure temporarily filled the vast space of the building's interior. This was the part of the whole operation that patient and rescuers would always remember, though Steve at the time tried hard to ignore it. Each metallic clunk announced that the metal mass was a little higher, but was an intimidating sound for the two beneath. The ambulanceman could feel his wet shirt clinging to his shoulder blades as a stabbing sensation streaked the length of his left arm, which still supported Noel's back. Dave watched with concern as his colleague sweated it out. During this operation he was unable to help; his partner was on his own.

It took several minutes to raise the weight to an acceptable height and then the cranking noise abruptly ceased. While Steve remained in position the rest of the rescue team prepared for phase two of the operation. As soon as the police crew returned with O-negative blood, Mr Phillips commenced an immediate whole-blood transfusion. He then retired and spoke aside with Dave Rees. 'OK, the patient is entirely in your hands now. The method of removal is up to your people. I wouldn't have the vaguest idea where to begin.'

Dave spoke briefly with the Hillingdon crew. Ambulanceman Graham James had just completed treating the lad's fractured leg with sterile dressings and an air splint, and he was confident that the immobilisation would cause no problem in the removal. Using a rubber pillow, triangular bandages and an ambulance fracture board, the team took the first step of reinforcing Noel's spinal area. It was only now that Steve could withdraw his aching arm, which had been static for nearly an hour. It was almost light blue, and there was little feeling in his hand or arm. A sturdy lightweight alloy frame, called an orthopaedic stretcher, was made ready. This device separates into two parts and is normally reassembled underneath a casualty, but it could not be used like that on this occasion. The only practicable method was for Steve to support the lad from above while his partner did the same from below. The Hillingdon crew, while helping Steve, would take care of other essentials during the transfer.

Dave removed his tie and squatted beneath the patient's body. The move across was going to be a problem. Lifting his sticky palms above him, he gripped the fracture board and pillow, which were now under Noel's back for support. Dave shouted his readiness, as three pairs of hands steadied the lad from above, prepared to act on the word of command. 'Go,' barked Steve, and the four ambulancemen acted in unison, applying all their strength in a cautious manoeuvre that took them only half the anticipated distance.

'Hold it,' came from Dave, below; he had the most difficult job. Craning his neck to one side, he repositioned himself and clutched the board tightly for a second time. On the word, the team eased the patient aside once more—now only inches from the stretcher. A final motion brought him firmly on to it. Steve stood up to stretch his aching muscles. He felt light-headed, and his legs needed brisk movement to bring life back to their dormant muscles. His arm still appeared discoloured as its circulation slowly returned. Looking ahead his eyes caught the blank expression of Noel's father, who waited uneasily.

The orthopaedic stretcher was gingerly lifted and placed on the red-blanketed trolley-bed of Hillingdon 1, Noel covered with a pre-heated shock blanket and strapped to the trolley bed for safety. With the infusion bottle firmly in the theatre technician's grasp, the patient was carefully wheeled to the waiting ambulance. Dave stood aside as the Hillingdon crew took over. He strolled over to his partner and offered him a smoke. Steve did not need coaxing, lifting the cigarette to his dry mouth with slightly trembling fingers. 'Are you going to see the father or shall I?' Dave asked as he held out a match. Steve cupped his hands about the flame and inhaled deeply. He would tackle this.

As the Hillingdon vehicle pulled out of the compound, two-tone horns trumpeted ahead from the police escort. The local traffic division had organised a problem-free journey, with police control at all intersections. Watching the ambulance disappear into the rush-hour traffic was the lad's father, who turned to face Steve for the first time: 'How is he?' The ambulanceman paused and chose his words with some deliberation, torn between truthfulness and the need not to upset the man more than he must. 'He's broken his leg, and injured his back. These are two of the obvious problems, together with a swollen abdomen. He'll need some surgery, but to what extent I can't say. There's no telling what the end result will be . . . I can only hope with you.'

The man thanked him and walked away with some of his colleagues, past the dispersing fire appliances. 'Thanks, lads,' Dave shouted across to the group of helmeted firemen, who nodded as they replaced their equipment. Steve and Dave wandered back to their vehicle, to sort out the chaos inside, apparatus lying on the trolley-beds and the floor. Control called through, and Steve reached for the microphone: apparently a vital medical case had been left behind on scene and was required urgently by the hospital. Dave spotted it tucked under one of the beds: someone in the factory had probably picked it up in an effort to be helpful and placed it in the wrong ambulance. 'Roger, Red Base, on our way; ETA five minutes.' Without further discussion, Dave closed the back doors and climbed into the driving-seat, joined by his partner who stared at his paperwork. Their blue-grey uniforms were highlighted by yellow streaks from the half-painted piping.

Steve himself felt sick as the ambulance glided into the street, not because of bodily discomfort but from his state of mind. He had come to know the trapped patient on a personal level, sharing the same uncertain danger throughout the rescue operation. He now felt that he had lost contact with a friend, and a general emptiness filled his mind as he tried to revert to routine matters. At Hillingdon, it was not practical for the crew to see the casualty, but they learned that he was to undergo immediate surgery before being transferred to an intensive therapy unit.

A week later he was sent by ambulance to Stoke Mandeville Hospital outside the London area. Although his other problems were overcome, he was left with permanent paralysis below the waist. Both Steve and Dave had expected that this would be the outcome, but it was still hard to accept for someone so young. As months elapsed and many had forgotten the incident, Steve decided to go to see how Noel was getting on. Personal involvement with a patient is frowned upon in any sector of the medical profession, but to deny a simple human emotion would perhaps be worse.

The Stoke Mandeville Hospital, specialising in spinal disorders, can be a sad place for the outsider looking in. Yet the patients themselves have remarkable energy and zest for life, a commitment to accept the worst and try to make better what they have. When Steve arrived at the bedside he was greeted instantly; even after three months Noel had not forgotten the ambulanceman who had treated and consoled him at the warehouse. Steve found it difficult to know what to say and could only admire the lad who had been but a few weeks away from starting a university course. Now much rethinking had to be done and a new start made; Steve could not help wondering what he would have felt if he was now in Noel's position, but he could not picture the prospect for long.

Steve Manhire and Dave Rees are still in the Ambulance Service. They continue to work as a crew and have tackled numerous cases in various predicaments and situations. Since choosing their line of work they feel they have made startling discoveries about the world, society, people and themselves. The 'metal block' incident gave Steve a greater insight into his own personality. His concern for a fellow human being in the line of duty led him to risk his life. Few people have the chance to test and understand themselves in this manner. Ambulance work is one of the jobs where such a situation may occur, and when it does the realisation and self-evaluation are totally unexpected.

2

Making the Grade

A 'grade 4' ambulanceman, who bears the distinctive laurel-leaf motif on his left shoulder, has reached the standard of training and experience required to begin his career. It will have taken him a year, but he is still considered 'wet behind the ears'. Of every twelve people who apply for a position as an emergency ambulanceman or woman, eight will be interviewed and only two accepted for training. There is, of course, no guarantee that either of these two will pass the comprehensive course of lectures, practicals, exams and field training: it is a career that does not at present require formal qualifications but instead sets an entry exam. Why is the percentage of people accepted so low?

The very nature of ambulance work demands a certain type of individual, with personality, common sense and the ability to keep a cool head and professional manner at all times; someone who can apply the deft skills required to deliver a baby or perhaps remove a spinal-injury patient from the murky depths of a London sewer. The right bedside manner, a pleasant and friendly demeanour, are vital when dealing with the sick and injured. This extract from an article entitled 'What is an ambulanceman?' is taken from the July/August 1977 issue of *Ambulance Journal*, with the editor's permission.

Not a doctor But we must make a diagnosis based on history, signs, symptoms; decide a course of treatment to stabilise or maintain the patient's condition, or decide when definitive treatment overrides the need for diagnosis, ie cardiac respiratory arrest.
Not a nurse But we apply nursing techniques in ambulance nursing to ensure correct patient positioning and comfort during the journey.

Not a social worker   But we are often approached by people suffering hardships or see hardship, such as old people without heating or adequate food, poor living conditions, neglected children, and in consequence advise appropriate departments.

Not a midwife   But we on occasions have to deliver babies at home or in the ambulance, or in environments not suitable to us, the mother, or the baby, because Mother Nature dictates when and where.

Not a policeman   But we must understand road traffic law, the law in relation to forced entry, the law in relation to restraint, Public Health Act law in relation to forcible removals, and the complexities of the mental health laws.

Not a fireman   But we must understand and apply rescue techniques in crash situations, knots and lashings, effects of toxic loads, and precautions, the toxicity of our own fire extinguishers in relation to our patients' conditions should the need arise to use them.

Not a mechanic   But we must practise basic mechanical knowledge in the event of breakdown, either to rectify faults or pass back information to mechanical sections.

Not a sociologist/psychologist   But we must deal with people in their sub-cultures in stress situations, which affect attitudes, and know the acceptable standards of behaviour in that particular culture.

Not a manager   But we manage a situation, plan short-term, utilise resources and man-power plant available to achieve a stated objective efficiently, and manipulate the environment to reach the objectives.

Not a physiologist   But we must be able to identify the effects of G-forces upon the injured or defective internal organs caused by the various changes in direction and braking of the vehicle.

Not a racing driver/chauffeur   But we must travel at high speed, yet be able to give a slow comfortable ride when required.

To this extract I would add some definitions of my own:

Not a clerical officer   But we must document all cases.

Not a navigator   But we must guide our partners through strange territories, reading the roads correctly under the stress of serious emergency call-outs.

Not an entertainer   But we must improve a patient's sometimes bleak outlook on life, entertaining sick children and keeping their worried parents reassured.

Not an anaesthetist   But those of us who have advanced skills must introduce air tubes into lungs and enter veins to administer fluids and certain drugs when needed.

Not a physiotherapist   But we must encourage and instruct certain patients to use their limbs correctly especially after strokes and other crippling ailments.

Not a diplomat   But we must be careful how we deal with every situation especially in other people's homes or in the public eye.

Not a mental welfare officer   But we must be aware of the uncertain nature of patients with mental illness; how to manage them efficiently and have the ability to see beyond their present state of mental disarray.

People from every conceivable walk of life apply for ambulance training: plumbers, bus drivers and 'clippies', librarians, medical technicians and nurses. Nowadays there seems to be a trend for graduates to apply, and I myself left a teacher's training course in favour of ambulance work, joining the Ambulance Service with a view to temporary employment, as I had plans to study for a place at medical school. When I realised that my new job was so interesting, demanding and unpredictable, plans for a university place were eventually discarded.

My career with the Ambulance Service began on a brisk spring morning at Divisional Headquarters, The Mall, Kenton. As I ascended the stone staircase of the large building, behind me were 'front-line' crews, busy attending to their ambulances. Much as I wanted to become one of them, I just could not see myself being accepted. At nineteen years of age, I had little experience of life and no experience of working in the outside world.

A cloud of smoke hung like a blanket above the heads of the six other candidates in the interview room. I remember the smartly dressed woman who puffed nervously, tapping her foot uncontrollably against the magazine table in the middle of the room. She twitched at me with the side of her mouth. I took this to be a smile and returned the gesture. 'Oh God, I wish they'd hurry up.' She lit another cigarette from the smouldering butt of her last one. 'Been waiting long?' I enquired, trying to make conversation. 'Not really, love, I've done my written tests and I've just got the driving test to go.'

She inhaled deeply, expelling the cigarette smoke slowly through her mouth and nostrils. The door swung open, and an officer in crisp white shirt and epaulettes stood in the doorway, holding a clipboard in front of him. 'I'll take the lady next,' he said cheerfully. My new-found acquaintance stubbed out her half-smoked filter-tip into the ashtray that looked like a mass grave for fallen dog-ends. 'My name's Madge,' she whispered as she rose to her feet. 'It's been nice knowing you.' She reached for her handbag and walked out, followed by the ambulance officer.

There was a deathly silence now in the all-male gathering. Each interviewee sat with his own thoughts. I looked at them in turn, trying to fathom out what their ages and backgrounds might be. The average age seemed about thirty, although one candidate was about my age and, at the other end of the scale, one man was about forty-five.

It was not long before I found myself in an exam room, and a feeling I was used to but never relished swept over me. The test papers were placed before us, and I slowly worked through them. The questions were much harder than I had anticipated, and some demanded a lot of thought. Following this came a verbal memory test, and then we were back in the waiting area for another ten minutes.

My driving test was perhaps the greatest ordeal of all. A Mr Garrett called me out of the room and led me downstairs to an ageing ambulance, which looked almost pre-war. 'Jump in Mr McCoy. Right then, let's see what you can do.' I had already been warned that this test vehicle had a 'crash' gearbox, which entailed double-declutching through the gate. I took a deep breath and started the engine. My nerves were only now becoming noticeable. I revved the engine a little and glanced at the examiner as if I wanted a round of applause. 'Carry on, Mr McCoy.' 'Oh, right,' I said, pretending I was waiting for his command all along, and then I made my initial attempt at getting the first gear. A ghastly crunch, which must have set the poor man's teeth on edge, was followed by several other assorted rude noises, and I eventually selected the gear. I depressed the accelerator and released the clutch, gripping the steering wheel tightly and leaning forward in anticipation of movement. Nothing happened and I increased the engine's revolutions. 'I think you'll find the handbrake useful,' remarked the officer in a calm, helpful voice. I swallowed, feeling my face become warm with increasing embarrassment. Reaching down, I released the handbrake, and the vehicle lurched forward kangaroo-like, smoothing out as we turned left from the station forecourt. Second gear seemed almost impossible as I clutched, double-declutched and treble-declutched. How I got the vehicle into fourth gear I can never remember.

After I had spent about ten minutes crunching around the neighbourhood and attracting odd looks, Mr Garrett asked me to stop the vehicle. This, I thought, was to be the depths of my embarrassment: he was surely going to tell me to walk back! 'Mr McCoy, slide over into my seat and let me show you how to handle this antique heap.' The last phrase lifted my gloom considerably. As if we were gliding on air, the officer breezed the old ambulance back to the ambulance station and reparked on the forecourt. 'Easy when you know how.' Yet I could barely return his smile. I felt that the end had come for me sooner than anticipated. But then I could hardly believe my ears: 'You've passed, by the way.' I looked at the examiner in amazement. 'I can see you have road sense and you can drive. Shame about the crash gearbox, but all our vehicles are automatic nowadays. You'll be OK in one of those. Cheerio.' I did not even return the farewell, such was my astonishment as I went upstairs once more. Before I could reach the door another officer summoned me for the final hurdle, the official interview. I smartened my tie, suddenly feeling that I was really in with a chance. I had to get this job. With a prayer on my lips I strode into the Divisional Officer's office and took the seat offered to me.

A Mr Jones sat at the desk before me. He had a pleasant manner about him and attempted to put me at ease. 'So you've passed your driving test,' he remarked, peering over his glasses, 'only nineteen too.' The Divisional Officer sat back in his chair and looked directly at me. 'So what makes you want to be an ambulanceman?'

I answered without hesitation since I had expected the

question. 'The work interests me; it's more challenging than teaching with more responsibility. A chance to work with the public out of the confines of an office.'

Little did I know that the answer to that question alone decided my suitability there and then. Had I said anything about blue lights, two-tone horns, blood and glory, I would have been shown the door. After a further twenty minutes of brief questions and answers, I was asked to remove my student-length hair in due course, attend a medical and, all being well, report in a month's time for training at Waterloo Headquarters. I was in!

Three months and many lectures and exams later, on an October afternoon, the big day arrived.

I felt nervous. My system seemed to vibrate as if charged with 240 volts, and I perspired profusely about my forehead. Admittedly, the second symptom was the result of a dash from the underground station to Ambulance Headquarters, the effort made in order to be in good time for my first-ever shift as a qualified ambulanceman. I had successfully completed months of study and exams at the Training School, which had included a spell at St Thomas' Hospital, and a two-week advanced driving course run by the Ambulance Service on police lines. I had been put through films, lectures, demonstrations, operating-theatre observations and maternity delivery suites; I had been shunted and hurtled about a skid pan, and lowered from the side of a building in rescue training. I now felt about ready to put some of this newly acquired knowledge and experience to some practical purpose.

Many ambulancemen would have said that at nineteen I was far too young for the job. The point had been raised at the initial interview when the examining board questioned whether my maturity was sufficient to undergo the training and subsequent work. It was not as if I had been an Ambulance Cadet from the age of sixteen. Nevertheless, I had been accepted, and had successfully reached the required standard before the twelve-month probationary posting. Right now I had to undergo at least six months operational training, mostly under an experienced training supervisor.

I entered the operational training station through a reinforced-glass swing door, and the warmth of the building rushed to absorb the sweat on my brow. I glanced at my watch, which showed 14.51; the duty began at 15.00, which gave me a mere nine minutes to calm down and get ready for this longed-for occasion. Both the ambulances were out— Quebec 1 and 2—so I made my way to the watchroom. Knocking on the door, I pushed it open cautiously. An officer in a white shirt, his back to me, faced the window, engrossed in reading a file. I placed my holdall down on the highly polished floor with an extra thud to announce my presence once more. The man at the window turned around and peered at me across the room. Feeling I ought to say something, I informed the officer who I was.

'McCoy? Welcome Mr McCoy. My name is Miller, your training supervisor. I have just been reading about you in a report here. You seem to have done quite well in the classroom.' I smiled, pleased by the remark. However, his next comments soon changed that. 'It means little, Mr McCoy; let's get that straight from the start. Your theoretical knowledge is very welcome, but it's strictly experience that will save life. Understood?' I was taken aback by the matter-of-fact approach and stood still, almost as if to attention. Then the training supervisor changed his tone.

'Now don't get me wrong, I'm not saying I look down on you for doing well upstairs. On the contrary, but I do want you to understand from the very onset that it's your direct practical ability that will help you sustain life, not the knowledge of how many ccs of blood are pumped through the aorta every second.' I remained silent. 'By the same token, I still expect you to keep up with your anatomy, physiology and basic medicine. It will form the basis of your practical knowledge.'

Not knowing quite what to say after all this, I accepted his invitation to sit down. A young woman appeared at the door, and I recognised her as one of my colleagues on the course. I managed to raise a controlled smile, still feeling uncomfortable in the training officer's presence. 'Ah, Mrs Taylor?'

'Yes sir, Helen Taylor.'

'Right. Take a seat next to your new partner, Mr McCoy. You are obviously acquainted. Now we have four minutes before you are on duty. While I have a word with your colleague, would you, Mr McCoy, take this key and find your locker. It's number 13—I hope you're not superstitious.' I picked up my belongings and went to the locker room.

By 15.10 my new colleague and I had begun our first vehicle check, making great efforts to carry it out exactly as we had been taught. We refrained from talking to one another on a personal level but exchanged glances and smiles as we got on with our task. I was rather cursing my luck, however: there had been only one woman on the course, and why did I have to work with her? Would she be able to cope when the chips were down? Could she carry a heavy patient competently? Similarly, I was later to discover, Helen was concerned by my youthful appearance, feeling that I was still almost a schoolboy. It had not worried her in the classroom, as she never dreamed that she would have to work with me. After the vehicle check, Helen and I introduced ourselves to the other training crew on duty, two more raw recruits but much older, about thirty. Roy and Keith had a woman training supervisor, Mrs Evans, a stout woman of about forty, greying at the temples, looking a warm, friendly person with an amiable charm.

The kettle was boiling in the messroom and six cups were ready to be filled with the first pot of tea for the shift. At the Training Station the messroom and watchroom were combined. There was no television as the senior training officer insisted that trainees were there to learn how to become ambulance personnel not film critics. Tea was poured, and our training supervisor agreed this was only to be a short break before we got down to some practical lessons in ambulance aid.

Before I could take my second sip of tea, however, the red phone rattled urgently. I went rigid at the sound and began to tremble slightly. Helen placed her cup on the table and stood up. Mr Miller had already reached for the phone and was taking down the call. He signalled to Helen. 'Come on, this is your job.' A wave of excitement, fear and nausea swept over me as, swallowing hard, I looked for my cap and buttoned up my jacket. The other crew showed some signs of uneasiness, realising it would be their turn next. Mrs Evans smiled reassuringly. 'Don't worry, just keep a cool head.' I appreciated the encouragement.

In the next minute it seemed as if all hell had broken loose. The noisy automatic doors were swiftly opened, revealing a fresh afternoon breeze outside. Helen and I hurried to the vehicle, unsure of ourselves. Miller looked at us in turn. 'Now, Mr McCoy, you should be driving, but I want you to sit in the attendant's seat for the first call. Helen, you sit in the back and observe from the front bench-seat through the cab door.' Neither of us was in a fit state to drive! My tremors increased as if someone was poking my legs with a bunch of pins. I tried hard to conceal my agitation, but the more I did so, the worse it became. 'Right, seat belts on. Helen wedge yourself in. We've got a "collapse" call. Someone has fallen and is possibly injured behind locked bathroom doors.'

I cannot begin to describe the thoughts that ran through my mind. I imagined a ghastly situation—perhaps a man gasping for his last breath, gore everywhere, turmoil and confusion. How was I going to cope? My hands shook and calf muscles turned to jelly. With a pulse rate of over 100, and a pounding machine in my chest, I was almost ready to become a patient myself. Despite the extensive training, films, doctors' lectures, practicals and assessments, there was nothing to simulate the real thing. This after all was what the job was all about: experience.

There is a special technique in driving an ambulance on a call. Tremendous concentration is required when the speed limit is broken, for the chances of an accident happening are high. The driver's reflexes have to be sharper than normal, and invariably his blood pressure will increase and his heart rate will rise. Even the most experienced ambulanceman or woman handles an emergency run with extreme caution, rarely taking risks: an ambulance that threatens an accident is a hazard not only to the public and their property, but also to the crew and the patient that awaits it. Any foolish manoeuvre that ends in disaster would mean the loss of one's driving licence and consequently the loss of one's job, even though it was performed with good intent.

The training supervisor pulled the ambulance out into the street, started the blue beacon and dipped the front headlights. 'I'm driving because I'm going to show you how not to drive. Despite the image television films bestow upon us, I don't want to see either of you driving like this, *ever*.'

Miller thrust his foot hard down on the accelerator and at the same time firmly swung the steering wheel to the right. The ambulance careered to the right with a screech of the tyres, and the rear of the vehicle leaned over to the left as if it were going to topple. Helen gripped the safety handles tightly as she felt the pulse rising in her throat. I clung to the underneath of the seat with my clenched fingers, pressing my feet against the front of the cab floor and hanging on for dear life. A further sudden acceleration made the ambulance surge forward, and Miller pressed the button to start the two-tone siren, which echoed resoundingly in the cab and made speech among us impossible. The training supervisor increased the volume of the radio to compensate for the high-revving engine and the use of the horns.

Looking ahead, I saw we were rapidly approaching the main road. I felt very unsafe at this speed, though I noticed from the corner of my eye that Miller looked relaxed enough. Again without warning the steering wheel was spun violently, this time hard left, into a vacant gap in the afternoon traffic. Thrusting forward like a turbulent wave the ambulance, which was now in the outside lane of the dual carriageway, headed straight for a busy road junction. Glancing at the speedometer, Helen was amazed to see that we had exceeded the 30mph speed restriction by 28mph. The traffic intersection was now only 500 yards away. Managing to turn my head over to one side, I saw Helen closing her eyes and leaning backwards. With two-tones blaring unmercifully, the traffic parted as the green lights, now thirty yards away, changed to red. Purposefully Miller stood on his brakes as if with both feet. I felt my safety harness hug me tightly with a binding force.

'Are you all right back there, Helen? You seem a bit quiet.'

In fact she was unable to utter a sound, and Miller grinned. 'Right, enough of this.' Passing the intersection, Miller eased off the accelerator a little. 'How would you describe my driving, Mr McCoy?' 'Well, I . . .,' I began, but Miller interrupted. 'Like a maniac? Would that be a suitable description?' I managed a wan smile, appreciating the vivid lesson. 'In order to help people to save life,' Miller continued, 'we must respect our own. If we kill ourselves or others on the way, we can only be classed as hypocritical imbeciles of no value to anyone.' As we approached another hazard, he added, 'Now, this is how I want you to drive on an emergency call.' Using his traffic indicators, he pulled the ambulance over to the outside lane and then, to avoid a hold-up before the roundabout, carefully eased over to the 'wrong side' of the road, as there was little oncoming traffic. Driving steadily but briskly, he used the audible warning device and flashed full-beam headlights at drivers ahead. By careful manoeuvring and selecting a lower gear from the automatic transmission, the ambulance was upon the roundabout. Traffic from the right slowly stopped to allow the emergency vehicle to take priority. Miller raised his hand in acknowledgement to the drivers, reselected a higher gear and smoothly accelerated away.

'OK you two?' Feeling a lot happier and safer, Helen found her voice. 'They're quite helpful, aren't they.' 'Only if you gain their respect as a skilful driver, not a damn kamikaze pilot.' We turned off the main road into a council estate. 'Always turn off your beacon and headlights if you're responding to a house call. It doesn't startle the family if the patient is not seriously ill or injured, and of course it doesn't bring the neighbours out in their droves.'

Miller stopped the ambulance in front of the appropriate block of flats, and I grabbed the immediate-aid satchel. Helen scrambled out of the rear doors and joined me. 'Go on, it's number 30. Remember, it's down to you now; I've only come along for the ride.' Still slightly trembling at the knees, I located the door marked 30. Then remembering that I was not in fact the attendant, I passed the satchel to Helen and stepped aside. 'Thanks Glen,' she was sarcastic. With that I waited for her to knock. As she stood on the step she was imagining someone who had stopped breathing—no, worse—had a cardiac arrest caused by electrocution; or perhaps someone drowning at this very moment in the bath, choking and spluttering while we stood here motionless. Just as she was about to knock again, impatiently, the door creaked open and the frail figure of an old man stood in the darkened passage.

'Ambulance Service.' The man did not respond. He looked at the crew as if he was in a world of his own. His grey cardigan covered a yellow stained vest and matching long pants. His outer woollen coverings had gaping holes in the elbows and sleeves; his misshapen slippers were almost in shreds and appeared to have been placed the wrong way round on his feet. Helen ventured forward and immediately caught a smell that we would both later remember as typical of a geriatric household in need of personal care. The stench was choking, particularly as it seemed to include paraffin fumes. 'Come on Glen, let's check the bathroom.' We made our way up the narrow, modestly carpeted staircase, the rank, fetid atmosphere becoming increasingly unbearable. The landing was small and dimly lit; all the doors were ajar except the one at the end of the passage. Helen tried it, but it was locked. Knocking loudly she called to the occupant within and distinctly heard a voice, but could not translate the garbled words into a coherent message. I felt I ought to fetch Miller to ask for advice, but Helen stopped me. 'Let's not be defeatists already. I think we ought to force the door.'

Sensing that this was my task, I put my shoulder to it and managed to break in at the fourth attempt. I was concerned that this mode of entry might in some way further injure our patient, but fortunately this was not the case. However, the sight that met us inside the bathroom was far from pleasant. Helen, who worked her way in first, could not believe what she saw. In the dim room was a bath-tub filled with old newspapers and books on which had settled a layer of dust. The musty smell mingled with the malodour of an incontinent old woman, at least eighty years old, obese with long wiry white hair and pointed fingernails (Helen thought they would have made Howard Hughes look well manicured). In a brown-stained nightdress which may have originally begun its life as pink, she was slumped on the floor, her head against the bath-tub. She stirred as if awoken from a sleep and spoke a few words, which sounded like 'da de da'. Helen had to withdraw, as already she was feeling a nauseous sensation creeping from her stomach to her throat. 'Oh God,' she whispered meeting my face on the other side of the door. 'What's wrong? Is she . . .?'

'No, she's breathing, but she's in one hell of a state.'

As I took a look at the patient, Miller came up to see what was happening. 'How are you doing?' he asked. Helen looked lost but tried to show she was in control of things. 'The lady has collapsed on to the floor, but she's still breathing.' 'That's reassuring,' remarked Miller nonchalantly. Helen realised he wanted her to make a further assessment. It was then that she appreciated how useless her theoretical knowledge was without prior experience. Patients like this never appeared in the Ambulance Service textbooks. Miller brushed past and looked inside the bathroom. He returned to a position out of the way and said softly, 'OK, I think you'll not disagree that we have an incontinent geriatric. What else?'

'She's had a stroke?' Helen suggested. 'Right. Her breathing, erratic behaviour, partial paralysis of the facial muscles and, I assume, limbs on the left side of her body point only too well to a cerebral vascular accident. So we'll need a chair, one large blanket, a rubber sheet and plenty of inco-pads. Agreed?' Helen was pleased that we now had a course of action though was also a little disappointed with her part in our first call. 'Oh, and you'd better wear your white coats and disposable gloves—for your own comfort.' As we both began to scramble downstairs, Miller called to Helen: 'Mrs Taylor, I suggest you remain with your patient. Remember, I've only come for the ride. I'm sure Mr McCoy can cope with the equipment.'

Trying not to think about the smell, Helen moved back to the bathroom and attempted to open the door as wide as possible by slowly moving the woman's legs to a more convenient position. She scanned the old lady's face again;

she seemed as if deeply asleep, snoring through the side of her salivating mouth. Helen remembered for a moment that this woman was once her own age, youthful, happy and active. Now, after four-score years, she had come perhaps to the end of the road. 'Helen,' I called quietly from behind. I held out a white coat and a pair of polythene gloves. Appreciating that it was our first job, Miller began to set up the ambulance carrying-chair and preheated blanket on the tight landing. We manoeuvred our way round the old lady, with Helen taking up position behind her.

Our crisp white coats brushed against the green verdigris on the side of the WC as our shoes sank slightly into a dark spongy fluid lying on the bare wooden floorboards. Helen grappled under the woman's arms and with my help grabbed her wrists firmly; the old dear must have weighed at least thirteen stone. Now squeezed in the corner of the room, Helen was ready to lift and tried to remember her lessons on body leverage so that she did not injure her back in the process. I came alongside the woman, my back to the WC, and slid one arm behind her back and the other under her knees, thus also taking a position for correct lifting. At the agreed moment, we moved in unison. With a concerted struggle we placed the old lady on the rubber-seated chair and blanket firmly held by Miller. We were ready for the downhill journey, with the woman tucked in between the warm blankets and strapped into the chair.

'Hello? Are you there?' came a voice from downstairs.

'Yes?' Miller peered over the flimsy banisters.

'Are you taking her?' The voice continued. Miller looked at Helen as if to engage her in this further conversation. Taking the lead, as the attendant and thus in charge of the situation, she replied 'May I ask who you are?'

'Yes love, I called you—I'm Mrs Burgin's daughter.' We looked at this lady somewhat incredulously as she made her way up the staircase. She was wearing a fine blue overcoat with a fur collar, her hair newly and elaborately styled. She was well spoken and seemed to feel no embarrassment at the shabby, if not unhygienic, conditions her parents were living in. 'You'll be taking her to St Thomas' Hospital—it'll be easier for me to visit her. I only live around the corner from there.'

Helen glanced at Miller and saw his head move from side to side. The ambulancewoman took her cue. 'No, I'm sorry, we have to take her to the nearest casualty department, which will be the Westminster Hospital.' The daughter's manner changed. 'That's no good. How do you expect me to get there? I'll have to get my husband to take me in the evenings, and he won't like that one bit. He works late and may have to come home early.'

I glared at the woman and burst into the discussion. 'How can you be so callous? You leave your mother in these conditions and your only concern seems to be yourself!' I was stopped in my tracks by Miller. 'Right, dear, if you'd just let us get on with our job.'

'Well, I don't know,' huffed the woman, 'I've never been spoken to like that before. I've a good mind to report you.' With that she turned and tore downstairs, brushing past the elderly man at the foot of the stairs, slamming the door behind her as she left the house. Miller broke the spell and urged us not to stand around any longer. With Helen at the top of the chair and me at the bottom, we carried the pathetic lady to the lower passage. The old man took the crew's 'breather' half-way down as an opportunity to lean over and kiss his wife.

'We shall be getting the doctor and social worker to come and see you Mr Burgin. You may need a spell in hospital too! Don't worry, we'll take good care of your wife.' Not expecting a reply, we carried the patient out of the flat. The fresh air pushed at our faces with its sharp invigorating flavour. As Miller turned to close the door, the old man who stood behind it whispered 'Thank you.' The training officer gave him a reassuring look and gently tugged the door closed.

It was customary and beneficial to discuss completed cases with one's training supervisor. Miller refreshed us on all aspects of cerebral haemorrhage, its implications and treatment. Eventually, he tackled me about my outburst. 'Our job is to care for and treat the sick and injured. We don't decide the rights and wrongs of the situation surrounding the incident. It is not our concern. At no time do you lose your temper with a patient or any one else for that matter. Understood?' I nodded. 'You're an ambulanceman, trained to keep a clear head and unbiased opinion at all times. Would you slate an unmarried girl for becoming pregnant or subsequently having an abortion? Of course not. It's none of your business.' 'Do you think she'll report me?' I bleated sheepishly. 'Oh, probably.' I looked worried. 'To the hospital—but, as you know, we're a separate entity and the hospital staff will not be in the slightest bit concerned with such a petty complaint. They'll probably tell her exactly what you did!'

Within the first months of operational training I was to observe casualties of a different kind—from within the ambulance station. Each week at least one ambulanceman or woman would leave the service for one reason or another. One had undergone a bad night shift during which he had witnessed three people die. He had been unlucky but could not endure much more of the incomparable misery he experienced in dealing with such cases. It had started with a suicide attempt that succeeded en route to hospital (the young patient had leapt under the wheels of a double-decker bus); then followed a fatal road accident in which an eighteen-year-old youth had been knocked from his motorbike into the path of an articulated lorry, which had consumed his body unmercifully; but worst of all was a baby that had choked on vomit, dying in his arms before arrival at hospital, despite his frantic efforts to resuscitate it.

Another trainee on my course booked sick and eventually resigned after his first resuscitation attempt. The case took place outside Trafalgar Square underground station, when an elderly man had collapsed with a heart attack. During the ambulanceman's rescue attempts, he resorted to basic mouth-to-mouth resuscitation while his colleague collected vital equipment. The act resulted in the inexperienced trainee forgetting to place something over the casualty's mouth first, with the subsequent consumption of ejected vomit. Other trainees left because they were unable to cope with the detailed paperwork between calls or with driving under conditions of stress or pressure. A colleague on my course 'wrote off' a brand-new ambulance when he jumped red traffic lights on an accident call. Forgetting his basic training, charged with excessive amounts of adrenalin, he failed to proceed through the stop signals with caution, and when he met a speeding saloon coming the other way, the outcome was obvious. Fortunately no one was seriously injured, but one man's career in the Ambulance Service was short.

Others leave the Service because of the effects the work has on their personal lives. Some find the great stress involved has indirect ill-effects upon their families. Wives dislike the long shift hours, which can ruin family life, and some ambulance-men even take their work home with them, waking in the night with bloodbath nightmares. For many, the long hours, low wages and excessive stress become too much. It is an unfortunate fact that the Ambulance Service has a high rate of coronary thrombosis among its staff. Others resign because they feel too much is expected of them. An ambulanceman is often faced with making decisions that he would rather avoid; yet he is compelled to make them because there is no one else to do it for him and no time to take the matter to his superiors.

One case I recall vividly concerned an experienced ambulanceman who worked in the West Country. He responded to a 999 call given as 'child difficulty breathing'. Needless to say, the crew did not waste any time in getting to the address given, arriving within four minutes; the address was not far from the Ambulance Station. The attendant leapt out of the cab and hurried to the open front door of the semi-detached home. From behind the door a trembling mother suddenly appeared, her long hair partly covering her tear-soaked face as she held the blue-faced, limp body of a young girl in her arms. Too shocked even to scream, she gasped to the ambulanceman; 'Please do something to save her— please.' Grabbing the three-year-old, he placed her on the hall floor. He could see from her now near-crimson ap-pearance that she had stopped breathing. So, checking that the girl's mouth was clear, he pinched her nose and pressed her jaws. Tilting the small head back, he took a deep breath, gently but firmly expelled warm air into the infant, scrutinising the child's chest. Nothing was happening. He tried again with no success. The ambulanceman realised what the problem was and, with his pen-torch and right index finger, probed deep into the dying youngster's throat while his partner raced off for oxygen and suction apparatus. With one hand on the girl's neck, he could still detect a faint pulse and his fingers met an obstruction deep in the throat. It was definitely immovable. Unfortunately this incident took place before the days of intubation (by which the entrance to the windpipe can be clearly located, and any blockage removed with forceps).

A decision had to be made—and fast. A rushed journey to the nearest hospital, at least ten minutes away, would undoubtedly be pointless. As the ambulanceman gripped the head of the child whose life was slipping away before his eyes, he decided on the only course open to him. No one else in the world could at that moment advise him. There were merely seconds to spare before the child's heart would stop and all be lost. The only chance was a technique he had never performed before; something certainly not taught to him during his training, but only talked about unofficially and read of in medical magazines. This was an emergency tracheotomy, which consisted of making an incision in the windpipe and then blowing air through it to the lungs. Complications arise if the incision is made in the wrong place, and the ambulanceman knew he was taking a big risk, but also knew there was nothing else he could do.

As his colleague returned with the equipment, he took out a pocket penknife and selected the long, thin metal punch on the tool, holding it forward in readiness with one hand and using the other hand to feel for the 'correct' place to introduce the instrument. He ignored his partner's plea and subsequent verbal barrage advising him not to do anything 'stupid', made a small hole and inserted a sterile catheter from the suction apparatus between his shaking fingers. Quickly he breathed through the tube and observed the wonderful sight of small lungs inflating. Within seconds the facial colour had altered and the pulse became stronger. The child was alive and soon began breathing on her own.

The mother cried with happiness on the way to the casualty unit. The casualty staff were a little taken aback by the sight of an emergency tracheotomy, but although their initial reaction was one of surprise, the duty houseman soon appreciated the situation. He could see that this was indeed the only action open to the ambulance attendant. The next day the casualty doctor telephoned the Chief Ambulance Officer to commend the life-saving technique he had witnessed. Within two hours the ambulanceman in question had been summoned by a superior officer, questioned about the incident, reprimanded for applying a technique he was not trained to perform and summarily dismissed.

In other emergency services, such as the Fire Brigade, men are trained to work under the direct command of an officer, who is present on the fire appliance at all times. Ambulance staff, however, are trained to work independently, decisions and responsibilities resting squarely on their own shoulders. It is a precarious position, sometimes proving too much of a challenge even for the most experienced people.

3
Call Red Accident

Strategically placed in every ambulance station in London is the all-important 'hot line', which serves as a direct telephone link to the Central Ambulance Control in Waterloo, south London. Along its extensive network originate the details of every incident in which human life may begin or be extinguished. In between these two extremes is a vast spectrum of situations, many of which will affect people for the rest of their lives. Apart from administrative details, these lines rarely bring good news. Among routine calls come sorrowful cries for help and urgent pleas for swift action in a desperate crisis. Ambulance crews are called upon for such a wide range of tasks that it is impossible to predict what an eight-hour tour of duty may unfold.

Train incidents are not a daily occurrence, but they are frequent enough in the London area. Apart from major accidents, the commuter train running along its electrified circuit may often be stopped by a human projectile, sometimes purely by accident, sometimes as a deliberate attempt at suicide. In either case, regardless of circumstances, the same course of action must be taken to safeguard and treat the injured patient. Often this is easier said than done because of the real danger that threatens any would-be rescuer. It would be disastrous for a member of an ambulance crew to become a second patient during his efforts to free a victim trapped under the solid mass of a passenger train.

At 7 o'clock on a fresh February morning, ambulanceman Stuart Webb signed on duty. He had qualified as a grade 3 ambulanceman just before Christmas, and so was still a probationer with little experience. At twenty-one years old he was the youngest on his station and consequently had to contend with a lot of leg-pulling from older colleagues. This morning he was working with Alan Levity, whose regular mate was on leave. These two worked well together whenever they were made up as a crew and hoped that one day they could be assigned on a permanent basis. The day's work began as fairly routine. One maternity case—a woman in labour—followed by a geriatric patient with a severe stroke. At 8.45 the crew radioed in 'green' and available at University College Hospital, and it was then that it received the first 999 emergency of the shift. Stuart, who was attendant, heard the two words he hoped he never would, the phrase that haunted new recruits like some dreadful demon: the ambulance term for a patient under a train, 'One under'.

Full details were obtained on the air and read back to Red Base. Alan pulled out of the hospital grounds while Stuart activated the blue beacon and front flasher units. He sat back in the attendant's seat, his legs shaking, his spine tingling and his muscles tensed. Traffic was heavy, especially along the Marylebone Road, but the crew reached its destination within seven minutes. Two station officials confirmed that this was no false alarm—so the first of three possibilities on a call such as this had been discounted. There was little to choose between the two remaining alternatives. Either the victim had been completely consumed by the train's velocity, leaving behind a trail of unrecognisable human carnage, or he or she was still alive with injuries as mild as bruising or as ghastly as severed limbs. In the first case the crew would be expected manually to collect the human debris and place the remains in the plastic bags provided for such instances. Although this prospect is horrific, the second alternative is perhaps even more distressing: a severely injured patient in enormous pain who is very much alive and totally aware of his predicament.

Grabbing his satchel, Stuart stepped out onto the pavement and walked briskly towards the station staff. 'Yeah, mate, down this way,' one said casually. 'A bit messy, but she's still alive and in one piece. You know it's the third we've had this year.'

This sort of build-up did nothing to assist Stuart's mental

state, and he felt that any minute he too would need an ambulance. He tried hard to maintain the confident relaxed composure instilled at the Training School. As the group made their way down to the platform, Alan asked if the electric power was switched off but would not take a simple 'yes' for an answer. Official confirmation soon came from the stationmaster, allowing the crew to begin its difficult task.

A solitary tube train stood halfway into platform 3, all the passengers having been cleared from the area. A sixteen-year-old station worker ran towards Stuart. 'I can see her clearly from the other side mate. She's moving.' At this point the ambulanceman forgot his own concerns and jumped down to the lines, clutching his satchel. There, partially obscured by the wheels of the train, lay a woman thrashing about in pain. Meanwhile, Alan had returned to the ambulance for essential pieces of equipment, including hand-lamps and pain-relief gas. With the help of a station worker he piled them on a trolley-bed and together they wheeled the stretcher down to the platform.

Stuart removed his jacket and got on his knees. It was dark underneath the train and he shouted for a hand-lamp. Alan grabbed two units and sprang off the safety of the platform to join him. 'I'll crawl down to her, then pass me the lamp,' Stuart said. Moving forward into the dark cavity, he wriggled under the heavy metal chassis of the commuter train. Keeping away from the rails and near the centre of the track, he crawled towards the body, of which he could see only a mop of hair. The enclosed space and tense conditions made him perspire profusely, and this was increased by his fear that the current might still be around him, perhaps reactivated by accident. Beads of sweat covered his forehead and ran down into his eyebrows. Then he heard Alan's voice from the side of the train and saw his arm sliding through a small aperture, a hand-lamp gripped tightly between his fingers. Stuart accepted it carefully, his hands trembling.

Crouching, he concentrated the beam of light and could see his patient, a woman in her early twenties with long shoulder-length hair. She wore loosely fitting jeans and a denim jacket and appeared to be grossly underfed. Stuart hooked the torch above him from part of the train and, inching forward, clasped the woman's head gently. Slipping out a pen-torch from his top shirt-pocket, he checked her level of consciousness. The size of her pupils and their reactivity to light would tell him something about her medical condition. He spoke to her, but she rambled incoherently. Continuing to survey the skull, the ambulanceman noticed blood coming from the right ear. He double checked and reluctantly concluded that the skull might be fractured. This became more apparent as the patient began to thrash about, gritting her teeth and salivating from the sides of her mouth. There was also the possibility she suffered from epilepsy.

Trying to steady her, Stuart attempted to check for other injuries. Under the increasingly difficult conditions, he could see that, as well as facial lacerations, the upper part of her right leg was malformed, which indicated a severe break, but that her ribs appeared intact and her pelvis seemed normal. It was now apparent that he would be unable to administer pain-relief gas: the head injury was too serious—in these circumstances the gas would possibly harm her further. Getting her out of this predicament was going to be extremely difficult.

Suddenly the young woman's whole body locked rigidly. Stuart guessed what was about to happen and shot his hand into his jacket pocket to retrieve a plastic airway tube that he always carried for quick use. Wrenching impatiently at the sterile packet, he released the airway and pushed it into the patient's mouth. Her teeth were clenched fast, and Stuart knew that this would be the onset of a convulsion or seizure. He needed to insert the airway between her teeth to prevent her biting her tongue and obstructing her breathing.

Suddenly she gasped, and Stuart seized the opportunity to plunge the airway between her teeth. She bit hard, her jaws relocking into place as her face reddened. The ambulanceman grabbed her shoulders and forced them down in an effort to steady her, as her whole frame began to vibrate. After thirty seconds, as if released from the grasp of some unseen force, the woman's body relaxed once more, and Stuart heaved a sigh of relief.

He heard Alan calling to him to explain that there were two possible ways of extracting her from under the train: the train could be jacked up, which would take some time, or it could be driven off, which would entail re-electrifying the rails. Stuart gazed at the woman's face and battered body. He could see that her condition was deteriorating and that she needed immediate hospital treatment. As far as he was concerned there was only one course to be taken. The train had to be driven away.

Although the concentrated effort was beginning to make him feel light-headed, Stuart knew exactly what he had to do. Alan passed him several triangular bandages, and Stuart bound the patient to protect her. If she had another fit while the train was moving, it was more than likely that she would be electrocuted. 'You're going to come out of there, Stuart?' he heard Alan ask.

He paused. 'No, mate, I don't think so. She may break loose and get fried.'

'Yeah, but so might you if you're holding on to her! Come on, you're not expected to do all this.' Alan knew that he would probably do the same under the circumstances, but he felt he had to give his partner the option to come out. Stuart reached up to retrieve the hand-torch, which he placed near him on the ground. The woman's level of consciousness was still unpredictable even though she was bound like an Egyptian mummy. Stuart leant all his weight forward to try to prevent her moving. Alan gave the warning: 'They're ready, Stuart. Don't touch any of the rails!' Stuart knew that only one rail carried the current but was not able to find out which one it was. He hugged the woman, waiting for the giant machine above his head to move. Closing his eyes, his mind flashed back to how he had got into this situation in the first place: only eighteen months ago, he thought, he had been a trainee chef.

The train-driver waved from his cab, then the train moved. The sound of the machine snapped at Stuart's eardrums with sudden force as he grit his teeth and held on to his patient. Slowly the wheels of the train began to turn as metal ground against metal. As the train continued to back off the woman began to convulse again. Fear gripped Stuart's heart as his fingers tingling with cramp. Gradually the dark, sombre shape of the train was replaced by the bright neon lighting of the station. Stuart opened his eyes to several anxious faces peering from the platform, but he remained motionless, realising the continuing danger. Finally the all-clear was given, and Alan and the stationmaster jumped down to the track. Stuart was helped to his feet by his colleague; the uniform covering his aching body was hardly recognisable, covered with soot, filth and blood.

This was by no means the end of the case; in effect, the crew's task had only just begun. The patient needed urgent treatment, which could be begun in the ambulance. Red Base was alerted while Stuart worked hard. A police traffic crew, which had been at the station during the rescue, offered to escort the ambulance to University College Hospital. The ambulance drove steadily from the station entrance into the London traffic, Alan trying to keep the ride steady to help Stuart. They arrived at the hospital casualty department in five minutes.

The following day, local papers featured the story halfway down the front page. Stuart gazed at the headline with disbelief and dismay: FIREMEN RESCUE WOMAN FROM UNDER TRAIN.

The young woman was treated for several weeks in the intensive-care ward but never regained consciousness. She had a long history of anorexia and depression.

There are times when an ambulanceman may be recognised for taking a risk—although this seems to be the exception rather than the rule. The following is a report of a similar incident.

On 20 October 1979, Mr F. P. Nye, an ambulanceman of Hackney Ambulance Station, in the North East Division, was called to the westbound platform of Bethnal Green Underground Station. On arrival, the patient, who had attempted to end his life by jumping under a train, was still alive and trapped in the pit under the rails below the fifth carriage.

Once the power supply had been switched off, Mr Nye, together with a police constable, climbed down under the train and administered aid, but was unable to remove the patient due to the lack of clearance between the train and the platform.

They both agreed to remain with the man while the train was moved, a distance of some 100 feet.

It was necessary to re-connect the power supply, for about three minutes, during which time the man struggled to reach the live rail in order to cause himself further injury. In addition to this, the movement of the carriages created a great deal of noise and showers of electrical sparks from which all were in danger of being burnt. The man was then conveyed to hospital suffering from multiple injuries.

Mr Nye, who joined the Service on 16 January 1978, behaved under difficult and trying circumstances in a manner which indicated more concern for the wellbeing of the patient than his own safety and upheld the best traditions of the Service. I also have pleasure in informing you that Mr Nye is to be awarded the Royal Humane Society's Testimonial on Parchment and a recommendation has been sent to the Home Office for the Queen's Commendation for Brave Conduct.

Accidents involving children are always upsetting. So often they appear to be the result of thoughtlessness, negligence or mere folly. From birth, children are susceptible to choking, convulsions, overdoses, falls and drowning. Often accidents could have been avoided if someone had used some commonsense in the first instance. Cot deaths are common and most of them are due to a cause not fully understood, probably some form of infection; the term 'cot death syndrome' is the only medical explanation in many cases. Yet occasionally that is not appropriate. At 9 o'clock one evening, I witnessed the lifeless body of an infant, and soon discovered that the mother had fed him at 3 o'clock, put him to bed and not checked him again until 8.45 that evening. She said she never bothered as he was so quiet! She had obviously never heard of the danger of regurgitation and asphyxia.

So many things left lying around the house are a great temptation to small people. The youngest drunk patient I have ever dealt with was five years old: together with his seven-year-old friend, he consumed half a bottle of Martini, a small bottle of rum and some table wine. Both children were practically unconscious, coming round only to vomit profusely. I felt sorry for them—they were only aping adults.

Child abuse always attracts outside attention far too late. It is the ambulancemen who are faced with the final and irrevocable outcome of an adult tormentor's work. Dealing with the battered, scarred remains of an adult is hard to face, but the savaged body of a helpless child will always prove too much for even the most experienced ambulance crew. It is this type of call that makes them wonder if they are in the right job or if they have had enough of the stress of ambulance work.

The 999 calls that are pleasant, to an experienced crew, are those to maternity cases, when a baby is born without problem in the house or ambulance. My first BBA (baby born on arrival) was traumatic, however, not so much for the mother as for myself! In 1974, when barely twenty, I received a routine emergency call for a woman in labour. With my then regular colleague Graham James, I was stationed at Greenford. The call was in Northolt, and it took us seven or eight minutes to get there. A young man was standing barefoot on the path of his house, wearing only a T-shirt and jeans. He shivered as I approached. 'Quick mate, she's having it!' I had heard this statement many times before but it never had amounted to much. Fathers-to-be often panic. 'Don't worry,' I said nonchalantly and followed the husband up the stairs. I smiled as the young man took them two at a time, not realising that this was for real.

In the front bedroom I could not immediately see the patient, who was obscured by the door. After the chill of the night air, the warmth of the room hit my face. But as I glanced around the door my colour drained and heart-rate quickened. There on the bed, with her legs wide apart, was a young woman in labour, clinging helplessly to the bedclothes. Between her legs sprouted the head of her first child. She grimaced uncomfortably. By now Graham was behind me, also surprised at the situation, although he had already had his first delivery some time ago and was at an advantage. 'I'll get the gear and radio for a midwife. Shout if you need any help.'

Before I could take him up on his kind offer, he disappeared, taking the husband with him. I gulped and took a deep breath, offering a nervous look of self-assurance to my patient. 'OK, dear, don't worry, just take it easy.'

I hurriedly removed my jacket and put on the surgical gloves, sent by Graham via the husband. I approached the bed and gently reached out to support the baby's head, which was continuing to emerge. I could feel the woman staring at my face between contractions, and I knew almost by telepathy the thoughts that were running through her mind: 'What was a young man who appeared barely out of school doing in this situation? Did he really know anything about midwifery?' I tried to engender a little confidence—made difficult by my shaking legs. 'Don't be concerned, I've done this sort of thing before,' I quivered. Just then, a further contraction brought the entire head out with a gush of fluid. The idea of a new individual being brought into the world by my own hands suddenly removed all my nerves. This would be a moment I would always remember. In a firm voice now, I was able to instruct the mother. 'Don't push too hard now; take things gently, the baby looks good.' Within twenty seconds the baby girl had emerged fully. I carefully turned her upside-down to drain excess fluid from the nose and mouth, and then, as if on cue, the infant unleashed a healthy scream.

'Lovely pair of lungs,' I commented, relieved and quite pleased with myself, as I watched a beam of delight creep across the mum's face on catching sight of her daughter. I reached for the maternity pack and removed the surgical clamps, which I snapped in position along the cord as I had been taught in Training School. I never thought I'd have to use them so soon. Placing the baby in a sterile blanket I tucked her snugly with mum.

I was surprised to find that Graham had been behind me for some time. He smiled approvingly and told me the midwife would be here soon. 'I can see you've done this sort of thing before,' whispered the mother. 'If only she knew,' I thought.

Since that time I have attended several other births, one actually taking place on the top of a number 83 bus. The mother was on her way to the hospital after getting pains while out shopping. London Transport acted with its usual efficiency and cleared the bus while a 'clippie' comforted the patient and we were called. Some crews have even come across babies who were born down lavatory pans before they arrived. During frequent contractions the mother has felt the need to visit the toilet, and the infant has had a rather wet delivery. Probably the strangest case I know of was that of a fifteen-year-old girl who gave birth prematurely in the night, entirely on her own. It was a great surprise to her and a shock to her parents. Bizarre as it may seem, neither the girl nor the parents even knew she was pregnant. They attributed her recent weight increase to her eating habits!

The motor car is the cause of a large proportion of ambulance work. Yet, of the vast number of traffic accidents (RTAs) received as 999 calls by Control, only a small percentage are fatal. Many are slight knocks and there are no casualties, while in others patients suffer shock and bruises but nothing too serious. They are the lucky ones. Heart-attack and stroke victims sometimes lose control over their vehicles and crash into walls, other traffic or pedestrians. Drunkenness also contributes to the statistics, with innocent motorists often involved. Bad and careless driving perhaps cause the remainder of such accidents, and some drivers do not stop to ask questions after a collision.

One dreadful incident occurred on Argyle Road in Ealing several years ago. A driver knocked down an old lady on a zebra crossing, and in his attempt to escape, and so avoid prosecution, reversed and hit the poor woman a second time; until then I had never appreciated the meaning of the word 'callous'. That driver is probably still on the road today, for the police were never able to trace him.

My first major RTA after being posted out of the Training School occurred during a night shift. The accident happened on the fast stretch of road approaching the Target roundabout on London's Western Avenue. It was a Saturday night, just after closing time, which may have had some bearing on the case. We had left a residential estate where our last case had been a 'refused aid'—the patient had declined ambulance treatment and transport. Red Base had instructed us to return and we were heading down Greenford Road towards the station. It was a busy night, and not surprisingly we heard our call sign on the air.

'Greenford 1, Red Base, Greenford 1, over.'

'Greenford 1, over,' I responded.

'Your position, please.'

'Greenford Road, approaching station.'

With that we were issued with a 'call red accident'. Details were exchanged, and John Robson, my partner on that occasion, who usually worked at Park Royal Station, accelerated fast towards Western Avenue. Control asked us to report on arrival. The accident sounded serious, and people were reported trapped in one of the cars.

The line of cars at the Greenford Roundabout shuttled to the side of the road as they heard our two-tone siren approach. John flashed his headlights aggressively at drivers who did not seem to react; they probably had their car radios on at full pitch. Leaving the roundabout, we moved up Western Avenue, and as we increased speed past the Kensington roundabout a bright orange glow met our eyes: a mass of shooting flames were lighting up the night sky. Three cars had been involved in the accident, one of which was on fire. The burning car had hit a concrete pillar off the main highway, then a second vehicle, which stood close to, but untouched by, the neighbouring fireball. A third saloon was neatly parked on the dual carriageway and appeared to have only minor damage, as if 'clipped' by one of the other vehicles.

As we drew nearer we could see the faces of several people standing around the blaze in a trance-like state. John parked the ambulance alongside the third vehicle and leapt out with a fire extinguisher, which he directed at the burning mass. I radioed through for Fire Brigade assistance and dashed down with my attendant's satchel. Before I could get far, John shouted back for a crowbar, and I hurriedly obliged. He had found that there was no one in the burning vehicle but that there were two seemingly unconscious people in the second car. I raced down to my colleague, who had more experience than I, and offered him the crowbar. He threw the spent fire extinguisher into my hands; it had not fulfilled its task, and the car still burned.

'I don't think the petrol tank's gone yet,' John shouted. 'There's two in the other car—stand clear.' He had already tried unsuccessfully to open the doors of the saloon. He raised his hand, clutching the crowbar but, just as if a grenade had been tossed in our direction, the burning vehicle's petrol tank exploded. Flames shot skywards as the petrol ignited. I could feel the heat biting into my cheeks. I blinked hard, brushed away the grit that had blown its way into my eyes, and looked back at John who was ready to have another go. The rapidly approaching two-tone siren announced that the London Fire Brigade would be here soon. Nevertheless John pressed on, as we were not even sure whether our patients were breathing. Several blows with the crowbar were needed to shatter a side window before John could reach inside for the door handle; but the door still would not move. With a lamp I peered in at the occupants of the car. The torch lit up the shadows cast by the flames' glow, and I was able to make out the shapes of a man and woman. Since I am slightly built, it occurred to me that I could probably crawl through the window, and helped by John I slithered into the vehicle feet-first, trying hard to avoid the people's heads. Sliding over into the back seat I raised the driver's head. The car was so hot that I felt as if I were in a sauna bath, and the stench of stale alcohol met my nostrils. The man, whose head I held in my hands, was breathing all right and could be easily roused if shaken hard. I eased his head back as he slumped forward in a drunken stupor. Raising the woman's head, I was a little taken aback: her face was bright red and her eyes were staring; she was vomiting, and I soon realised what was wrong: her airway was obstructed. Shouting to John for suction apparatus, I somewhat reluctantly plunged my index finger deep into her mouth, extricating what I could, and compressed her abdomen sharply.

When John returned with the sucking plastic catheter, I plunged it into her mouth until I eventually heard the obstruction shift, consumed by the hungry little machine.

The patient gasped, then vomited violently. I could feel my arm soaked as streams of fluid ran up my sleeve.

It did not take long for the Fire Brigade to remove the doors from the car, and since they had no apparent injuries, we did not object when two burly firemen carried the couple in one of their well-known lifts. I for one was anxious to wash my hands. The stench lingered about me uncomfortably.

It was only when we returned to the roadside that we discovered who was the driver of the now burnt-out car, whose grimy shell lay smouldering. Sitting in a police car was a middle-aged Chinese, who declined hospital aid, saying he had only suffered a bruised knee. He explained how he had been forced off the road by a lunatic driver. Time and time again in my job I have seen the innocent suffer.

With all the unpleasant cases described in this chapter, you would think that the average person would appreciate being in good health. Yet in the Ambulance Service we frequently come across people who deliberately attempt to put their own lives at risk—as a half-hearted bid for attention, or as a serious move to end it all. The most common method is an overdose—but this is usually for the amateur or those intent on being rescued in good time. Exhibitionists bent on creating a public scene dangle themselves precariously over high-rise balconies or threaten to jump from suburban bridges into the murky depths of polluted waterways. A small proportion succeed, making no mistake about their action. These are the people who hang themselves, leap off tall buildings without an audience, lock themselves in garages to inhale the poisonous fumes of a car exhaust, or drench themselves with petrol and burn themselves alive as human torches. These people we pity, for they are desperately distressed and perhaps if someone could have talked with them they might have been saved. I remember dealing with a case in Greenford where a fifteen-year-old schoolboy hanged himself in the loft for fear, it was later surmised, that he was homosexual.

Recently a crew from my station were confronted with an individual in what is, perhaps, the smallest category of all: that of those who do not want to die, but are prepared to take the final step if pushed that bit too far. Earlier this year, a crew from my station—Doug Wright and Bob Malham—was called to a council estate near Greenford. The call was passed over as 'a man threatening suicide'. When they arrived on scene, three police cars stood casually parked outside the terraced house. Bob, who was attendant, was met by a friendly sergeant: 'We've got a right one here; saved it for you special!' Doug asked what was going on. The officer explained that a middle-aged man had spent the afternoon busily banging a hole through his ceiling. Bob looked puzzled, and the sergeant signalled that they should come in and see for themselves. At the top of the second staircase, they turned into the living room, nodding to the policeman who stood outside. As they went round the door, their gaze fell upon two more policemen, craning their necks to peer through a gaping hole in the thinly constructed ceiling. One constable glanced in the crew's direction and smiled wearily. Bob moved forward and looked through the opening, through which he saw, sitting on a beam, his neck encircled by a stout rope, a man in his late forties; his ruffled appearance seemed to match his state of mind.

Bob looked at the rope carefully. It was neatly tied in true cowboy fashion, and as his eyes followed it upwards he realised this man meant business. The end of the rope was tied securely and neatly around a wooden beam near the entrance above. One of the police officers took Bob and Doug aside and explained the situation to them, asking if one of them would like to make contact. Bob volunteered. He stepped on the coffee table that had been placed beneath the opening and called to the man. 'Who are you?' grunted the voice from above. 'I'm just an ambulanceman,' returned Bob, trying not to aggravate the situation.

'What are you here for? I haven't jumped yet,' reasoned the man, almost jokingly. 'How about coming with us to the hospital? Come and talk it out,' Bob answered. The response was: 'Why don't you all piss off and leave me alone?' Bob retreated from the table. He soon became aware of a plan the police had hatched. He noticed a large sheath knife with a thick wooden handle tucked behind Doug's back, and when he resumed his position on the table he was joined by a constable. Their two heads stretched towards the dark interior of the attic. Bob re-established communication, speaking quickly to try to gain the man's undivided attention. The policeman chipped in with the odd word of agreement.

Doug cautiously moved behind the policeman, keeping the knife flat against his back. The officer surreptitiously accepted the instrument, and suddenly lurched forward with unexpected force to slice vigorously at the secured rope. This sudden manoeuvre startled Bob, even though he knew it was to happen. He saw panic cloud the man's face before he grabbed the severed rope with both hands and dashed to the other side of the loft. The police officer saw him re-attaching the lashing to another beam and guessed what he would do: 'Get me up! Get me up!' he yelled, and Bob, Doug and the other police officers tried to heave him into the loft.

As they scrambled to lift the policeman, the noosed man plunged forward to the surface of the thin ceiling that separated the loft from a bedroom underneath. He plummeted through the wood and plaster with a crash, scattering debris over the carpet. His feet smacked hard on the floor, his knees buckling at the force of the impact. The well-harnessed noose tightened around his neck. The police and ambulancemen raced along the corridor to the bedroom, bursting through the door to find him choking, his beetroot-coloured face darkening with each passing second. While the sheath knife was put to work again, Doug helped support the man's weight and Bob darted off for his resuscitation pack. However, when he returned he could see that his colleague had brought the patient round; normal colour was returning and his breathing was regular.

'It's lucky these houses are all built a bit cockeyed,' said the police sergeant. 'Matey here obviously forgot that his bedroom floor was a little higher than the floor in his living-room. If it hadn't been, he might have broken his neck.'

Tackling the wrath of an uncontrollable fire is not the task of an ambulanceman. Such an awesome job is best left to the highly trained firemen, who give a superb service. Nevertheless, there are occasions when an ambulance crew is first on the scene of a fire and is obliged to take immediate action. On many occasions crews have rescued people, having to put their own lives at risk, especially as they do not wear protective clothing. Fortunately such incidents are few, since the Fire Brigade always responds promptly. But I remember one fire that was particularly upsetting. It happened on a caravan site in Northolt. We were given a fire call to an unofficial encampment just off the main dual carriageway where a caravan had caught alight from a paraffin heater. The black clouds of smoke hanging malevolently in the sky guided our approach. No fire engines were yet on the site, and I radioed Red Base to ascertain that they were on their way. Uncontrolled panic and unparalleled horror met my eyes. A woman screamed from the side of the blazing mass. 'My children, for God's sake get them out!'

My colleague and I rushed forward. The two small fire extinguishers we carried were not designed for large blazes, and although we tried to direct them on the caravan door it soon became obvious that there was no possible way of passing the intense heat that seared our faces and hands. I stood back, shielding my eyes from the heat and particles of smouldering debris that floated above the inferno. Never before have I felt so helpless and confused, and all the time the screams of the hysterical mother rang in my ears. It is soul-destroying to be trained to save life and yet to be unable to get to one's patient, either to effect a rescue or offer emergency treatment.

One entire family died in a fire that spread like lightning through their house. Their mortal remains sat around in lounge armchairs as if they were totally unaware of what had happened, their lives taken with the speed of light.

Coping with severely burned victims is always a gruesome task. Those that are not seriously burned are, of course, in greatest pain, their still intact nerve-endings transmitting agony to their minds. The ambulance crew can do little for such victims, as the entonox gas carried has little effect. Plenty of wet dressings can of course remove some discomfort, with an intravenous infusion perhaps for severe cases, combined with special burns dressings. Burns cases following explosions add a further complication, as injuries are more complicated than burnt flesh. Priorities in explosion casualties may become difficult to assess and far more difficult to treat.

The most unusual victim of a fire I have had was a whippet, which had been left alone in a flat in Northolt. The poor dog hid under the bed as the fumes filled the small rooms. Rescued by a fireman, it lay at the front door, coaxed by a firefighter who could only offer air from a cylinder. We brought along some oxygen and tried this on the animal, whose respiration was fast and husky. It's true that children and animals in trouble always steal your heart. Fortunately the story had a happy ending. With the help of the police the dog was taken to an emergency veterinary surgeon who over a short period brought it to full recovery.

In all but a few cases it is an ambulance crew who will remove and transport a patient to a hospital casualty following a 999 emergency. At times, however, this is not a straightforward operation. In the following incident, the crew took six hours.

During a middle shift, Ambulanceman Lucas and Ambulancewoman Cottrell, a crew from Whipps Cross Ambulance Station, received a routine call at 16.00 hours. The case was given as 'female-neglect, ulcerated legs and verminous'. The crew selected a sparsely equipped ambulance to avoid contamination and put on special clothing. Arriving at the address given, the team was met at the door by a gentleman who introduced himself as the patient's brother. Explaining that they were in for a bit of a shock and a difficult time, he led the pair into the front room. The room itself was cluttered, and there were layers of dirt and dust across the mantelpiece, shelves and shabby floor. A ghastly stench filled the room, which had once, perhaps, been cosy and well-furnished.

Two 1930-style chairs had been placed together to create a make-shift bed, and there, on the 'divan', lay an elderly lady. Despite her state of health, the old woman managed to greet the ambulance crew. They discovered that she had slid down into a lying position over a period of time and that now both knees were bent and fixed awkwardly in one position. The crew established that their patient had been wedged in this position for three months without being moved anywhere— not even to use the lavatory. Although the poor woman had lost all track of time, she was by no means senile, though the attendant found her pulse weak and slow. Beneath the fetid blanket enveloping her, the woman wore nothing save an old top, stained with faeces and urine. Her knees, which had been resting against one of the chair arms, were now 'fused' to the vinyl covering, part of which had penetrated her flesh. The slightest movement caused her severe pain. Her weak condition was further complicated by arthritis, and the attendant suspected gangrene in the swollen, pus-ridden lower limbs.

While the attendant continued to assess the woman, the brother spoke to his partner, explaining that he was quite unaware of the severity of his sister's condition, although he realised that she had not moved for some time. It was, the brother said, only now that she had allowed him to summon a general practitioner who, in turn, had arranged for an emergency ambulance.

The crew's initial attempt at cutting around the vinyl fabric so that it and the woman's fused body could be moved had to be abandoned. The movement caused her too much pain, and there was also the possibility that the armchairs would disintegrate, they were so completely saturated. It was clear that further help would be required before their patient could be moved. Any severe pain could lead to a serious state of shock or a sudden haemorrhage.

The only conceivable way of removal would be to strap both chairs, together with the patient, on to a firm surface and then take the old lady out through the front-room windows. This manoeuvre would need the co-operation of the Fire Brigade and perhaps a casualty doctor to offer pain-relief treatment if necessary. While his colleague went to make the necessary arrangements, the attendant stayed with the patient, and even though she was in some pain, the old woman managed to share a joke and exchange a smile. While they waited the ambulance crew gave her some entonox gas and cleared the room of furniture. The floor was wet and had to be covered with newspaper to prevent anyone from slipping.

The Fire Brigade arrived at 18.00 hours. They were there on the strict understanding that they would work under the instruction of the ambulance team, which they were happy to do, and began by removing the lounge window-frame. From there, I can quote directly from the case report submitted by the attendant.

The Accident Unit Doctor arrived with his assistant and examined the lady. He agreed that our decision not to remove the lady from the armchairs had been right. She was in no condition to be subjected to anything that would cause her any undue pain and was not fit to be given an anaesthetic. She was quite relaxed and chatted as best she could to us. It was suggested by the doctor that photographs be taken of the room and lady by the Police before she was removed, because there was the possibility of legal proceedings being taken. This would cause only a slight delay and it was felt justified in the circumstances. The Fire Brigade also had a photographer with them who photographed the entire removal. The photographs were thus taken and by then the firemen had removed the window-frame. We were then ready to attach the ladders to the chairs. Next, the rest of the rubbish between the chairs and the wall was removed. This consisted mainly of newspapers and biscuit with urine soaked cheese wrappers. There were also maggots and mice under the chairs. When the ladders were securely attached, the fire, police and ourselves together as a team, lifted the lady through the window over the garden wall and into the ambulance.

The procedure had by now attracted most of the neighbourhood and there was some considerable interest being shown.

Ambulance Control and the Accident Unit Doctor had informed Whipps Cross Hospital of the circumstances and condition of the patient. They took some convincing that she was in fact going to arrive fused to the two armchairs. The journey to the Hospital was a slow convoy. The Accident Unit Doctor travelled in the Ambulance, his assistant following in a car. The police cars and Fire Brigade brought up the rear.

Time now 20.00 hours.

On arrival at the Hospital the Medical Registrar briefly examined the lady in the back of the Ambulance and suggested that two adjoining cubicles be made available in the Casualty Department. The chairs were lifted from the Ambulance, still using the ladders, and placed onto a hospital trolley.

It was decided that the chairs should be dismantled as gently as possible. The nursing staff removed all accessible clothing from the patient.

A draw sheet was passed between the two chairs and held ready as the arm chair supporting her head and shoulders was drawn backwards. This was replaced by a box the same height as the other chair. Thus one chair was removed completely. The vinyl covering of the remaining chair was now split to reveal the internal fixings. The bolts securing the back of the chair were removed and the back section then became free and so gently pulled away. The removal of this back section revealed a mass of maggots which had gathered down the cracks.

This caused the chair to be unbalanced on the ladder and so was re-positioned. In order to undo the side bolts the chair had to be lifted from the trolley. This was achieved by tipping it, using the ladder as a lever and holding the trolley down. A hand could then be passed under the seat to get to both sides of the bolts. The chair arm was not attached to the flesh and was thus removed.

The other side proved more difficult but the patient was eventually freed.

Five wooden boards, 3ft 6in × 9in, normally fracture boards, were pushed above and below in order to give firmer support. An orthopaedic stretcher (borrowed from another ambulance which arrived at the casualty during these proceedings) was then applied under the wooden boards with difficulty, and was refastened together. We now had the patient lying on her back on wet sodden soiled clothing and blankets on top of the fracture boards on the orthopaedic stretcher. Her knees required constant support.

The patient was soon positioned so the stretcher could be lifted and the lady rolled gently from one trolley to the other so that she became semi-prone on some sterile dressings.

This revealed her back to be one enormous pressure sore with several very deep areas of extensive pus with gross faecal and maggot contamination. The patient was now undressed on a trolley in the semi-prone position. Pillows were used to give extra support where necessary.

The nursing staff began to clean her with antiseptic solution.

Throughout her removal from the chairs the lady showed great patience and tolerance of the pain from which she must have suffered.

The time was now 22.00 hours.

We subsequently saw this lady on the ward and she was quite well and expressed her gratitude for everything that had been done for her. Although very sore she was eating well and looked much better. There were plans for her to receive physiotherapy to straighten her legs. There was fortunately no gangrene. She made very good progress for several weeks, but sadly contracted pneumonia following an influenza epidemic, and died six weeks later.

A follow-up letter from the accident unit casualty officer Dr Hindes to the Ambulance Service, read:

> Last Saturday I was invited by the Red Base Co-Ordinator to attend this incident and assist the ambulance crew with a difficult removal. Briefly, this was a case of gross neglect in which an elderly woman had been left in two armchairs pushed together as a bed for at least three months.
>
> My main reason for writing this letter is to acquaint you with the extraordinary nature of this removal, and to offer the highest praise to the Whipps Cross Ambulance Crew involved for their dedicated care of this patient for nearly five hours in the most offensive and foul conditions imaginable. I worked for several years in the East End and saw many infested vagrants, but I have never seen such a dreadful case as this.
>
> The ambulance crew had assessed the whole problem (and taken measurements to ascertain that she could be removed in the chairs on ladders to the ambulance), and the Fire Brigade who worked under their direction demonstrated an excellent example of team work.

Northwood Hills has always been regarded as a pleasant residential area, a large proportion of the homes belonging to the wealthy and exceptionally wealthy. I have found the work in this area most diverse, the cases being either trifling or extremely serious, with little in between.

One night shift, after a routine admission into the casualty department of Mount Vernon Hospital, my colleague Colin Sexton and I received a 999 call to an address in Northwood Hills. Only a house name was given, located in a private road that was unmarked on our map. A vague instruction about shutting the wicket gate after use accompanied the address. The actual call was recorded as 'a collapse'. I always become anxious when there is a problem in locating an address; I cannot help thinking of the patient who is waiting for urgent attention and whose condition may deteriorate meanwhile.

Colin was never one for hanging around when it came to a call or 'shout'. With his exacting, almost military, style of driving, he shot the ambulance smoothly out of the hospital grounds. The blue lights lit up the dim night sky; no horns were needed, of course, and indeed could not have been used at half-past midnight.

It was only by sheer chance and a little local knowledge of the area that we found the house, Red Base Control's offer to ring the caller back becoming unnecessary. The residence that matched the house name was an impressive sight, even with only the poorest light illuminating the large porch. We could see lights on the first and upper floors. I hastened up the gravel path while Colin parked the ambulance ready for a quick getaway before following me. The crunching of the stones beneath our feet seemed to carry for miles around in the desolate silence. Clutching my immediate-response satchel, I grabbed the large iron door-knocker and announced our arrival. The second tap eased the oak-panelled door ajar, revealing a slit of light and allowing some warmth to escape from the house. 'Come in,' called a woman's voice. 'The door's open.'

We lost no time and hastened into the plush hallway, which remained in semi-darkness, and followed the light source into a grand living-room. A central chandelier, sparkling like stars, lit the walls of the large room, which were covered with elaborate carvings and oil paintings in a variety of styles. An enormous open fireplace, the focal point of the room, had a small wood fire burning quietly in the grate. As I crossed the thick pile carpet, I almost felt that I should take off my shoes, as it was rather like walking on someone's bed, until my soles met the remains of a wine glass, which had been shattered across the path to the beautiful young lady who was sprawling elegantly across a leather settee, looking for all the world like an Arabian princess. 'Are you the patient?' I asked. She turned her head towards me and smiled faintly. Her dark blue evening-dress was covered with sequins, which glittered in the light of the fire. She could have been only five years older than my own twenty-one years. Long chestnut hair framed her face.

'What's the problem?' I enquired meekly.

'I'm so sorry to have called you out, but I had a dizzy spell earlier and felt quite faint. Now I've got the most goddam awful headache.' And she flickered a smile at me again . . .

'Would you like to come with us to the hospital?'

'Not really.'

Colin chipped in, having emerged from his observation of the room. 'Would you like us to get your own doctor to see you? We can arrange it.' She reflected for a moment. 'If you must.' She slid her feet into a pair of fluffy white slippers and stood up slowly. She swayed a little, holding her head, and I steadied her with an outstretched arm. 'Thank you,' she said politely and walked across the room. 'You'll find the doctor's number and name by the telephone, but unfortunately the line has been disconnected.' (Colin later discovered that the lead had been wrenched from the wall.)

'I'll use our radio.' Colin nodded to me and walked out.

'Can I fix you a drink, darling?' She turned to face me, a cocktail in her hand.

'No, thank you.' My reply was made through force of habit; I was captivated by this lovely creature. 'Shame. I hate drinking on my own.' She glided across the soft carpet almost as if on wheels and returned to the chesterfield. 'Come and sit down while you're waiting,' she continued, sipping her drink. I strolled over and pulled out a footstool in front of her.

'You ambulance people work odd hours don't you?' I nodded dumbly. 'What time do you finish today?'

'Oh, about seven o'clock this morning.'

'I don't envy you, I'd rather be tucked up in my bed.'

'So would I,' I replied, and then bit my tongue with embarrassment. She laughed and leaned forward towards me a little more. 'Can you guess what I do?' I paused for thought. 'A business lady?' She beamed. 'Well, sort of. Take a look at those magazines over there, the fashion journals.' I glanced at the cover of one with surprise: 'It's you!'

'That's right, they're all me.'

It finally dawned on me who it was I was dealing with, and I felt intrigued to be there. Yet before I could speak again, I saw tears forming in her eyes. 'My boyfriend has left me, you know. He walked out this evening.' I was a little taken aback by her direct approach but tried not to react too obviously. 'I get so fed up,' she continued, blowing her nose. Her wet eyes and tear-stained face did nothing to diminish her magic. Just then I felt my toe press against something hard in the carpet. I thought at first that it was a piece of the shattered wine glass, but closer inspection revealed an object of value. I picked it up and held it to the light.

'Oh, you've found it! I wondered where it had got to.' I was holding a diamond earring, and offered it to its owner. She clasped her hands about my outstretched fingers. 'Keep it; it's yours.' I could not believe my ears as she insisted I should have the diamond, and then she slowly pulled my hand towards her body. At last I snapped myself out of the trance; retrieving my hand and placing the earring on the coffee table, I stood up, adjusted my tie and jacket and walked towards the door. Colin came into the room as I was halfway to the door and announced that a doctor would be calling within the hour. He looked at my flushed face curiously. I bade goodnight to the woman, who had resumed her original position on the sofa, and led the way into the cool night air. I took a deep breath and felt like a cigarette, even though I normally did not smoke.

Colin sensed that something had happened and had to hear the full story. 'She must have been drunk to want you!' he declared, when I told him what had taken place.

'But just imagine, Colin,' I retorted. 'She was offering me money—and a whole lot more!'

There were no more calls that night, and I had plenty of time to think: my basic instincts as a man had battled with the conduct demanded by my job—a job that became more unpredictable with each passing year, and consequently more fascinating.

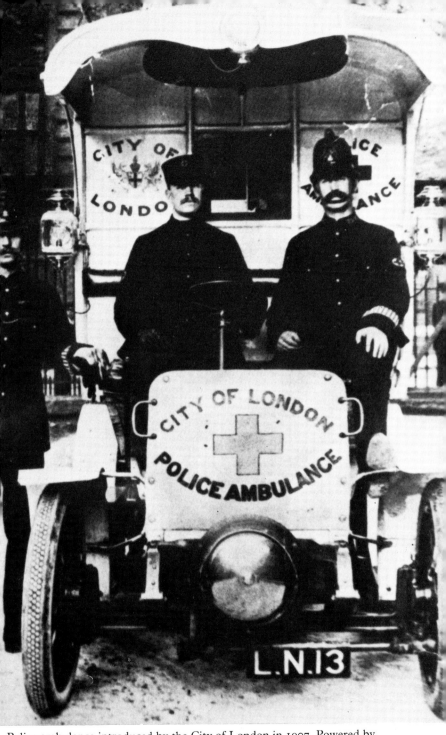

Police ambulance introduced by the City of London in 1907. Powered by electric motor, it was operated in conjunction with fifty-two call boxes (*London Ambulance Photo Library*)

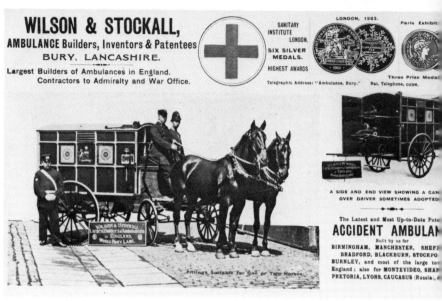

Early twentieth-century ambulance (*London Ambulance Photo Library*)

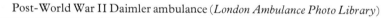

Post-World War II Daimler ambulance (*London Ambulance Photo Library*)

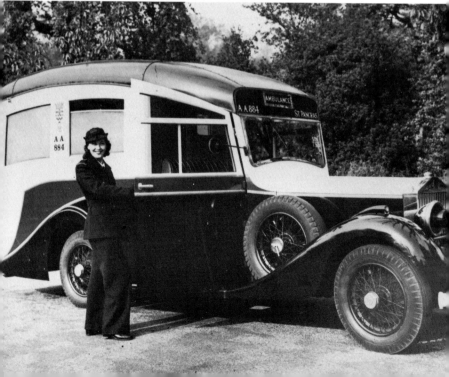

4

Meeting the Public

'Touch my collar, touch my toes, I hope I never travel in one of those.' I remember chanting this rhyme as a child whenever I spotted an ambulance. The sight of the white vehicle with its opaque windows that appeared to conceal some dire secret always alarmed me. Many people still take the same view, turning their heads away rather than catch a glimpse of what is perhaps considered an unlucky sight.

In big cities, however, ambulances are commonplace today, especially in London's West End and City areas, where the stresses of fast living produce many sudden illnesses, particularly cardiac cases. The two-tone sirens are familiar sounds to pedestrians, who see front-line crews contending with traffic conditions as if taking part in an obstacle race. The image of speed and urgency, underlined by flashing beacons and blaring horns, causes people to stop and take notice. Many mistakenly believe that this is all ambulance work consists of, but in fact 'blue-light work' accounts for 10 per cent of ambulance duties, and there have been times when I have worked four or five shifts in succession without touching the switch marked 'beacons'.

People rarely think of an accident ambulance as a mobile intensive-care unit in which a patient is treated and calmed down. It is rare for an accident victim to be hurtled to hospital on blue beacons and two-tones. Such extreme measures would only intensify his upset state of mind and possibly cause further injury, especially if he had fractures. Only serious cases of unconsciousness or cardiac arrest, and patients so acutely ill that death threatens, are conveyed rapidly to an accident and emergency department. Those who see the work of 999 ambulances in a different light have only the misinformed media to blame.

Just as the general public observes ambulance crews performing their public duties, so ambulance personnel study the various types of individual in society at large. We often see people behave rashly or erratically, sometimes with disturbing repercussions. This chapter looks at some occasions on which an ambulance crew's contact with the public has been far from pleasant if not extremely alarming.

People's attitudes to ambulance staff depend largely on their previous experience of the emergency service. Most of them appreciate what we do, but some complaints are made and for a variety of reasons. Some of the grievances are justified, and the crews concerned are disciplined. But some are less clear-cut. One complaint that I remember happened at the Richmond Ice Rink, a fairly frequent location for accident calls. An Isleworth crew was summoned to a fall on the ice, and found the patient to be a young lad of about seventeen who had suffered no more than a bruised knee; worse cases probably occurred at the local kindergarten where a kiss from the teacher would have been an adequate cure. Nevertheless, the crew checked the patient's graze and decided that the condition did not warrant specialised treatment. Although quite prepared to take him to hospital, they politely explained, they felt that it would be a wasted journey for the patient himself.

Suddenly an earpiercing yell came from behind the crew, who turned and saw a mother clutching an injured child, a little girl, whose condition, the attendant quickly saw, was quite serious. She had fallen and suffered a nasty skull injury. Without giving the matter much thought, the crew immediately took their new patient to the waiting ambulance and, after some ambulance aid, conveyed her to the nearest casualty department.

A few days later the crew was asked to attend a service disciplinary hearing at which it was confronted by the boy with the bruised knee. He and his family had complained that the crew had refused to take him to hospital. Despite the circumstances, the Ambulance Service had, reluctantly, to find the ambulancemen guilty of not conveying this 'patient', and a 'black mark' was recorded against them.

A similar situation occurred when a Greenford crew took a known heart patient to Central Middlesex Hospital. As they wheeled the fifty-year-old man into the accident and emergency department, he suffered a cardiac arrest. The team immediately began resuscitation and called for the hospital 'crash' team. In carrying out his duty, the ambulance attendant found it necessary to rip the man's clothing from his chest, tearing his shirt off and ripping off his jacket sleeves. After a ten-day spell in the coronary care unit, the man walked out of Central Middlesex feeling fine. A few days later, however, the hospital received a letter of complaint from the same gentleman who owed so much to his rescuers. He submitted a bill for the cost of replacing his ruined clothes.

Some thoughtless people in London appear to have no time or respect for the city's ambulances. An approaching siren seems to annoy them, to be designed to disrupt their busy lives. Needless to say, these people have never been in desperate need of an ambulance. Sometimes, when I have been travelling slowly with a seriously injured patient, I have been hooted at by passing cars; some drivers have even gesticulated rudely because of my deliberately slow pace. They do not seem to realise that the slightest bump in the road can make my patients cry out in agony. I suppose such misguided drivers assume that ambulances are supposed only to travel at breakneck speed. I am indifferent to motorists who raise two fingers in my direction, but I get angry with the ones who sound their horns and upset the already anxious casualty.

The junction of Perivale Lane and Western Avenue, near the Hoover factory, at Perivale, is a place where ambulances seem to be particularly prone to abuse. There is no right turn, but for the patient's comfort I often turn right here when it is safe to do so, rather than taking a long, uneven diversion. Unfortunately this does not go down well with some motorists, who seem oblivious to the vehicle I am driving.

Some road-users take things a stage further and refuse to allow me to pass. I quietly drift around those who genuinely 'freeze' when they see the blue repeaters in their rear-view mirrors, provided I am sure they are aware of my presence. But then there are the motor cyclists who will try and race me to the call. They become a threat to other road-users and a danger to themselves. Perhaps they get a kick from travelling so closely to an emergency vehicle, but I have yet to see them try this stunt with a police car!

Many people regard an ambulanceman as having a responsible, professional job, in which commonsense, medical know-how and experience are brought to bear on the range of problems that face him. Yet some still regard my uniform as that of a chauffeur, bus driver or general dogsbody. I once had a 999 call in Greenford to a teenager with severe abdominal pain. When I walked into the hall, a sixteen-year-old girl was sitting on the stairs, doubled up and apparently in great distress. I felt a wave of sympathy for her. 'Wembley Hospital, driver,' said the mother, as I was about to evaluate the patient's condition. I turned to the lady, forcing a smile: 'I'll just see what the problem is first, and then, if necessary, we'll go into the nearest hospital, which will be Northwick Park.' The patient leapt to her feet as if the pain had vanished completely. 'Take me to Wembley,' she demanded. 'I went to Wembley the last time!'

'I'm sorry,' I explained. 'Wembley is not the nearest hospital, and, in any case, it does not receive ambulance cases.'

With that the mother flared up as well: 'Then get out! We'll take a taxi.' Before I could utter another syllable, my colleague and I were firmly ejected into the cold night air and the front-door was slammed in our faces.

I have also found that relatives who travel with the patient expect you to drive them home from the hospital in the 'big white taxi'. Others have even stopped front-line vehicles in a manner which suggests they require emergency assistance, and then just asked for a lift home, insisting that they are a patient of some hospital or other. People's lack of understanding about what exactly the job entails is a problem that ambulance crews often encounter. Subtle offending remarks are delivered without malice but in total ignorance: 'I suppose you people must know a bit of First Aid.' 'You will stay with the patient in the back won't you?' 'How long have you been in the St John's?' 'I know your job back to front. I used to drive an ambulance during the war.'

Then there is the phrase that will delight any attendant arriving on the scene of a call: 'Get a stretcher!' (This comes even if the patient is on the top floor of a small narrow-staired town house.) People do not realise that carrying a stretcher about and conveying a patient are the last of an ambulanceman's priorities. The number one concern is 'How is the patient?'; the second is 'What treatment is required?'

All public incidents seem to attract a crowd, most of whom are nothing more than gawpers, revelling in someone else's misfortune. Once on Greenford Broadway, outside a baker's shop, I was dealing with an elderly woman who had broken her leg. She was in severe pain and greatly upset and acutely embarrassed by the contingent that had gathered to witness her sorry state. I shouted to people to move off, but no one took notice; in fact mothers actually pushed their children to the front so that they could get a better view!

During rescue operations for the massive air disaster at Staines in 1972, some rescue teams, including a fleet of ambulances, were hampered from getting to the scene for almost two hours. The path had been blocked by the hundreds of sightseers, armed with cameras and binoculars.

Gary Martin and Tony Moyle are two good colleagues of mine who work outside the London area, men I have known for many years. Their work always reflects their earnest enthusiasm for, and interest in, ambulance work. I shall never forget the events that led this crew to a particularly tragic call. Their faith in human nature was shattered through the malevolence of an adult. They were prepared to accept abuse and misuse of their services from society at large, but on this unforgettable shift a young boy's life was spent through thoughtlessness and blatant malice.

Wednesday, 16 August, 07.00 hours Control started the shift with the customary check to confirm that all vehicles were fully manned. Gary entered some details in the

Occurrence Book and returned to the messroom to join in the general chat. At 07.17 he and Tony, who were 'first out', started with their first job. The young ambulancewoman, Sally Jones, who was in the watchroom, jotted down the details of a call, tore the ticket off the pad and handed it to Tony, who peered at the diagnosis given: 'Sudden illness'.

'OK, see you later, Sal.' Gary had started Lima 10's engine and the crew left the station smartly. It took only four minutes to reach the address they had been given and Tony, as attendant, made his way up the path to a detached bungalow set between weeping-willow tress. He clutched his ambulance satchel and knocked on the door. After a second knocking, the door was opened by a man in his dressing-gown. He staggered a little, then sat down on the stool in the hallway clutching his head. Tony went in and knelt beside him. 'What's the problem?' He assumed the man to be the patient.

'I do feel rough.'

'Do you suffer with anything normally?'

The man seemed unsure. By this time Gary too was at the doorway. 'Did you call for us?' asked Tony.

'Yes, er . . . would you like a drink?'

'No thank you. Could you tell us why you might need our assistance?' The man looked at his guests, and Tony could see that his pupils were dilated. It was obvious that if the man had anything it was a hangover. 'I thought you'd be able to give me a good recipe for a headache.' Realising that their time was being wasted, Gary became flippant. 'Yes—a mallet, mate; excellent recipe for a headache.'

'Look, Mr Coleman, if there's nothing medically wrong with you apart from a hangover, we'll have to leave you to recover yourself.' Tony was irritated. 'I presume you don't wish to go to hospital.'

'No thank you son; just give me something for the headache.' The crew explained the position and their prospective patient eventually closed the door. They walked back to the ambulance. Tony completed his paperwork and radioed in to inform Control that they were available for further work. Control came through almost immediately with another call. It was an emergency admission, passed over by a general practitioner. 'Roger, that's from 117 Windermere House, Masefield Avenue. An acute appendicitis to the General at 07.48, Mike Hotel. Tango Mike.' Tony replaced the microphone in its cradle and began to write out the ticket. 'OK, Gary, go whenever you're ready.'

Gary gently accelerated away from the private residences and made for a large new council estate known as The Great Lakes, as all the blocks were named after large lakes. The estate itself was regarded as something of a vandals' paradise. Graffiti, mostly applied with felt-tip pens and spray paint, covered most of the walls, and the majority of roadsigns were badly defaced. Gary reflected on how he was once delayed getting to a cardiac case on the estate because he could not read the street signs. The delay did not help the patient, and it had been a close battle getting him to hospital in time. 'I get depressed when I visit this estate, Tony. I'd rather go off and live on a camping site.'

'Some of the people from here have done just that before now.' Ahead of the crew stood the tower block that they both knew was Windermere House although the nameplate now read 'ind rm   ous'. Gary parked the ambulance as near as he could to the main door, while Tony made his way to the unwelcoming entrance. As expected, the lifts were out of order, so he had to trek up five flights of stairs, wondering as he climbed if the patient was going to be heavy. The orange door of number 117 was covered with scuff marks as if someone had defied gravity and walked all over it. He had to knock three times before the door was answered by a teenage girl, who after seeing who it was rudely shut the door again. He heard her bellow: 'Mam! the ambulance is 'ere!' An older woman now came to the door, closely followed by a man in a car coat, presumably her husband. Before Tony could introduce himself, the woman gave her instructions. 'Me 'usband's following in the car, and me daughter's coming wiv me.' Tony, appreciating that the woman was the 'emergency case', asked her 'Are you in a lot of pain?'

'Nar, it's gone off now.'

'Will you be able to manage the stairs?'

'Yeah, I'm all right. Me 'usband's got a white van. Don't lose 'im, will yer?'

Tony assured her that the ambulance would not be rushing anywhere and led her to the stairs. As they emerged from the building he signalled to Gary that a chair would not be necessary.

'Who's the patient?' Gary enquired, before the woman and her daughter boarded the vehicle.

'Me, luv.' The younger woman took a seat in what was now all but a taxi.

'See you up the hospital, Jan,' shouted the husband, as he got into his van. Tony and Gary looked at each other, realising they could say and do little. All this had been arranged by a doctor. Closing the rear doors, Gary returned to the cab, and, at Tony's signal, the ambulance pulled away. Tony sat opposite his patient and asked further into her case. 'What did your doctor say when he saw you?' He was aware what was wrong with the woman, but on no account did ambulance staff impart medical information.

'He never saw me,' confessed the woman.

'Well, how did he arrange for you to go to hospital then?'

'Over the 'phone. I rang him this morning, told him I had a pain in the side, and he called for you blokes.' Tony shook his head but continued to complete his job ticket. Gary made good time in the early stages of the rush hour, and reached the hospital at 08.21.

They set out to return to station from the hospital, but today was busy. They were called up on route to go to a local school to deal with a child with a head injury. The Ambulance Service receives many calls from schools, although only a small percentage require a fully equipped emergency vehicle. They carefully made their way through the morning throng of blazered children to the main entrance. Tony was met by a man who introduced himself as the senior master, who told him 'You may need a stretcher.'

Tony politely delivered a stock reply: 'If you don't mind, may I see the patient first?'

'Right. What hospital do you come from?'

'Ambulances are not attached to hospitals,' Tony replied:

he was always surprised that people did not realise that.

'Oh, well. What hospital will you take him to?'

Getting a little irritated, Tony asked again: 'May I see the patient first, please?' The teacher, somewhat surprised at Tony's insistence, led him to the school first-aid room, where a middle-aged woman in a white coat was bending over a boy of about ten, bathing his forehead with a wet flannel. She looked round as the two men entered. 'Ah, ambulance, good. Which hospital are you going to?'

Tony did not answer the question but asked, 'What's the problem?'

'This boy fell over on his way to school. He's cut his head.'

Tony leant over the child and smiled. 'What have you been up to then, eh?' He gently examined the head. 'Was he unconscious at all?' he asked.

'No, he remembers everything.' Tony looked for a wound but could not see one. 'The cut you mentioned, where is it?'

'Just behind his left ear.' The woman pointed. Tony looked at the place and saw a thin red line, about half an inch long. 'Is this it here?'

'Yes, it was bleeding before you arrived.' The ambulanceman smiled but said nothing as the patient was only a child. He checked that this was the boy's only injury. 'OK then, we'll take him to the local General.'

The woman looked puzzled. 'I thought you'd take him to the other hospital in town? It's nearer, surely?'

Tony knew that she was incorrect, but he did not interrupt her. 'And I think it would be nearer his father's work,' the woman added.

Tony was firm. 'If you want him to go into town, may I suggest that one of your staff takes him there, as we only go to the General.'

The master entered the discussion at this point: 'Er, no, sorry, that's not possible, all my staff will be at assembly now; I've got no one to spare. That's why I called for you. I can't go breaking school routine.'

'You're absolutely right,' replied Tony, a little sarcastically.

The crew later learned that a little girl had been run over by a lorry and had had to lie miserably in the road for an extra five minutes because their ambulance, the nearest, was already committed to the unnecessary school call. The team that did eventually reach the child discussed the case with Gary and Tony and told them that the child had lost a great deal of blood and had been transferred to the intensive therapy unit.

The final call of the shift was taken by Tony at 13.58 hours. In fact the crew was already on the way to an urgent emergency admission, and had almost reached their destination when Control contacted them on the air to report their status. 'Already committed to your 13.52 call,' Tony replied. 'Child with severe asthma.'

'Roger, cancel your 13.52 call, take a further accident call.'

Assuming that another vehicle would be dealing with the asthma case, Tony took a new ticket and asked for details. 'Roger, it's a serious road traffic accident. Several patients reported. Query car overturned and now ablaze. We do not have a nearer vehicle.'

Tony scribbled down all the information and read back the call. Gary pulled out of the traffic and started the blue lights. The ambulance hurtled towards the reported incident. The asthma case meanwhile had been delayed until another vehicle was available.

The accident was supposedly at a new roundabout, half a mile outside the town on a spur road. Gary and Tony scanned the horizon but saw nothing. After several minutes, Tony called Control for further details but none were available. Control rang back the number given by the caller, and it turned out to be false. The call was malicious—a hoax. Tony confirmed the information and asked for new instructions. To his surprise, Control reissued the asthma call. 'Further information just received on the asthma case—boy going blue.' In dismay, Gary spun the ambulance about, and they sped along the fast stretch of road towards the address they had been given. Tony dashed to the house carrying basic resuscitation equipment, while Gary prepared the ambulance to receive their patient. He picked up the portable oxygen device and hurried to join his colleague. As Gary entered the hall he heard a woman crying in the kitchen. He went towards the sound, and when she saw him she screamed: 'Why did you take so long?'

In the living-room Tony had begun mouth-to-mouth resuscitation. The boy lay motionless beneath him. As the child was so young, Tony did not attempt intubation, the task of a paediatric physician. Gary brought the oxygen alongside and once the boy was on oxygen, began gentle cardiac compression on the boy's chest. His lips were blue and eyes wide open. The crew worked for four minutes with no response at all; they decided to remove the child to hospital, continuing resuscitation techniques on the way. The boy was laid on the mobile stretcher, while Tony, kneeling on the floor, continued oxygenation, suction of the throat and cardiac massage. Gary told the mother where they were going, then made one of the quickest possible journeys to the nearest casualty department, being especially careful not to swerve around bends so that Tony could work effectively.

Gary sent a 'blue call' via Control to alert the hospital, and as the ambulance reached the casualty entrance the medical team was waiting. He glanced back into the rear of the vehicle, but there seemed no sign of response to Tony's relentless work to save the boy's life. The limp body was soon into the resuscitation theatre where the hospital staff continued to fight for the boy's life, but eventually had to admit defeat. Tony slunk out of the theatre in a daze. Gary had temporarily disappeared, so he walked into the washroom. Alone, he felt a wave of emotion come over him, held his hands against his face and wept.

Contact with the public left a further scar upon two ambulancemen when they helped two colleagues at a super-market accident. A woman had walked through a glass door and had serious injuries. Colin and Jeff were day-workers on an out-patient ambulance coach which had been flagged down in the street. Colin, at forty-eight, had given up the stress of accident work three years previously, and Jeff was a twenty-two-year-old waiting for a vacancy on front-line accident work. It was the middle of the afternoon when a worker at the store, wearing the distinctive orange-and-white overall, rushed up to the ambulance coach and opened the side door. 'Quick, there's a bleedin' lady in our doorway.'

Colin was about to make the obvious joke but realised from the woman's expression that it was something serious. He bumped the coach up on the kerb and jumped out, while Jeff grabbed the immediate-aid satchel from the rack above the driver's seat together with a red ambulance blanket.

As Colin reached the shop's main entrance he perceived a middle-aged woman propped up in the doorway, her ashen face slanted to one side. Her black, fur-collared coat was splattered with glass from the smashed door, and she now lay on the entrance mat, supported by a metal shopping trolley. A small group of customers stood on the other side of her, some with groceries in wire baskets. A grey-overalled male member of the staff knelt by the woman, attempting to bring her around with smelling-salts. Colin took instant command; despite his lack of recent experience, his many years 'on the road' as an accident emergency ambulanceman came flooding back to him, and he stretched out his hand to make a preliminary examination of the patient. The severity of the accident was then revealed. A large pool of blood began to seep from under the woman's body, covering the light brickwork floor at an alarming rate. One shopper fainted.

Jeff leapt up to help, but Colin had other plans. 'Jeff! Stay here. We've got a problem.' Jeff could tell that something was dreadfully amiss by the urgent tone of his partner's voice. Their patient, in walking through the glass door, had sustained a serious injury from the heavy sheet of glass that inevitably came crashing down on her. She had partially severed the femoral artery in her left calf. Any arterial bleeding is serious, but the femoral artery is virtually the largest arterial vessel in the body, and the consequences of a break in its wall are usually fatal. A completely severed femoral artery normally gives the victim two minutes to live.

Jeff helped Colin rapidly to remove some of the woman's clothing in an attempt to locate the exact position of the haemorrhage. The shop's manager hovered over them but was ignored. 'Jeff, get help here fast—we want a paramedical crew to set up a drip.'

Jeff helped to reposition the woman, while Colin attempted to elevate the lower limb before applying a sterile dressing, and then ran off to the ambulance coach to radio for assistance. Ambulance crews are taught never to run, but this had to be an exception. The haemorrhage became more profuse as Colin applied direct pressure to the limb. This seemed to achieve little as his reddening hands fought to arrest the flow. Reaching for a triangular bandage, he attempted to tie a tourniquet as a last resort, realising that ambulance crews did not normally use tourniquets on the strictest medical advice.

'Excuse me,' the manager persisted. 'Shouldn't you be taking this lady away?' Colin had nothing to say. 'I have my customers to think about. You are causing a lot of distress and preventing shoppers leaving the store. This is the exit door, you know.'

Had the situation been less critical, Colin would have spoken his mind, but under the circumstances he confined himself to saying 'Too bad,' and turned his attention to the unfortunate woman. He removed the triangular bandage and continued to apply direct pressure to the site of the artery. He realised that the artery was only slightly severed; a completely severed vessel would by now have drained the patient completely. Nevertheless, the pressure in the artery would gradually cause a larger aperture for the blood to escape through. The woman's only hope was an immediate intravenous infusion to replace the blood she had lost and then a whole-blood transfusion at hospital. Colin checked her pulse as he continued to press against the limb. He broke open another dressing, then a third and a fourth, placing them one over the other. It was like dabbing a swimming pool with a sponge. The patient's face looked pale and lifeless; she was breathing, but only just. Colin helplessly wished he had the equipment of a front-line ambulance: oh for some surgical clamps, he thought, ideal in a situation like this. Jeff returned at last to say that an ambulance was on the way.

'Desperate circumstances demand desperate measures, Jeff.' Colin asked for a further large ambulance dressing, which he placed over the previous four. Kneeling on his left knee, he began to apply his weight on the surgical pad, even though the soft white material soon became red underneath. He was reasonably sure that the leg was not fractured, but even if it was, he argued, this was the only solution. Tremendous force is required to stop any arterial bleeding; if a major artery is damaged, the force required is excessive.

A stream of blood ran out of the shop entrance on to the paving-stones outside, but despite this, a middle-aged lady attempted to stride across both Colin and the patient. 'Do you mind, lady!' barked Colin, but received only an incurious glance.

The approaching sound of two-tone horns lifted Colin's spirits, and Gary and Tony were the crew who emerged from the emergency ambulance. Gary hurried up with an emergency infusion kit, and Colin told him that he thought the woman had probably lost about four pints of blood, half her total volume. In seconds, a drip was set up and running, and the haemorrhage was temporarily arrested. Jeff and Tony brought the trolley-bed from the ambulance, securing it as near to the shop doorway as they could.

The patient was eventually removed from the floor of the shop by the four ambulancemen and placed gently on the trolley-bed. Jeff removed the keys from the coach, realising that neither he nor Colin was in any fit state to continue their afternoon's work, and radioed through to the local ambulance control centre to report the latest situation. He and Colin were told to travel with the accident team and shower and change at the station. The police insisted on escorting the ambulance to the nearest casualty, and Jeff travelled with them so that he would not be in the way while Colin helped Gary in the rear of the ambulance. The two emergency vehicles left the shopping centre at 14.22, wailing their way to hospital.

Our job is for public safety and welfare, but all too often the public will hinder us and abuse our skills and service.

5
Tales of the Unexpected

The ability to cope with the unexpected is an essential quality in daily ambulance work. Sometimes the unpredictable can be alarming; sometimes it is dangerous; occasionally it can be amusing.

A few years ago a crew from West London attended a collapse call. Although they made every effort to reach their destination fast, it was unfortunately too late; the patient, who was seventy-nine, died at least thirty minutes before the crew arrived. In a situation like this the crew's duty is to console the relatives and to organise the diplomatic removal of the body to the nearest hospital casualty department.

It was past midnight when the ambulance pulled away from the small residential road. Mary Webb, the attendant, radioed to Control to report, as Mick Styles, her partner, drove to the hospital. Once there, he went to find a doctor while Mary completed her emergency call sheet. Soon the back doors swung open, and a casualty officer leapt into the ambulance, with a nurse close behind. He peered at the features of the elderly man, reaching for his ophthalmoscope, which he placed near to the deceased's eyes, humming to himself as he did so. 'I do believe this gentleman has passed away,' he declared eventually. Natural death is rarely taken seriously by the medical profession: the additional mental strain would probably be intolerable.

Mick managed a half-smile; it was the wrong time of day for humour. Mary passed the casualty officer her clipboard and the doctor scrawled his signature on the pink ticket. 'Now I'd be obliged if you'd stay away from here tonight,' the doctor joked. 'Nothing personal you understand, but I would like to get some sleep!'

'Do our best, doctor,' returned Mary, turning to the nurse. 'Is the mortuary open?' The nurse confirmed that porters were on duty; they had taken the victim of a fatal road traffic accident across some time earlier. 'Funny,' she remarked, looking at her watch, 'they should have been back by now.'

'We'll check.' Mary returned to her seat and Mick started the ambulance, spinning it sharply about in one manoeuvre and causing the tyres to screech a little on the tarmac.

The mortuary was some distance behind the hospital and was surrounded by trees. A single light shone from a lamp at one side of the building, and the crew were pleased to see that the main lights in the mortuary itself were switched on. Mick reversed the ambulance up to the main doors. As the crew disembarked and wandered to the rear of their vehicle, they could hear conversation coming from inside, punctuated, inappropriately enough, by bursts of laughter. 'Someone's having a good time,' said Mick, peeping through the curtain-less window. 'Just take a look.'

Mary leaned over her colleague's shoulder and saw four people sitting at a small table, on which stood two bottles of whisky and a pack of cards; clouds of cigarette smoke drifted about. 'They're Brahms and Liszt,' concluded Mick. 'All right for some.' Mary tried the door, but it was shut fast. She knocked hard and rattled the door knob. 'Come on, open up, we've got a customer for you.'

It was some time before one of the porters struggled to his feet, tilting his head to try to focus his eyes. He swayed to the door, patting the two card-players whose backs were to the doorway as he passed. The fourth 'maverick' beckoned the ambulanceman to join the card school. Eventually the mortuary door creaked open and the ambulance crew walked in, a little taken aback by the party. 'Sorry to interrupt the fun, lads, but could we bring someone in?' Mick stared at the drunken porter who was attempting to return to his seat. 'Have a drink first!' shouted the second man, raising his glass awkwardly. Mick strolled forward, beginning to lose patience, and as he neared the drunken porter, he was grabbed firmly by the arm and pulled towards the table.

'Just look at my hand,' the porter exclaimed. 'But not

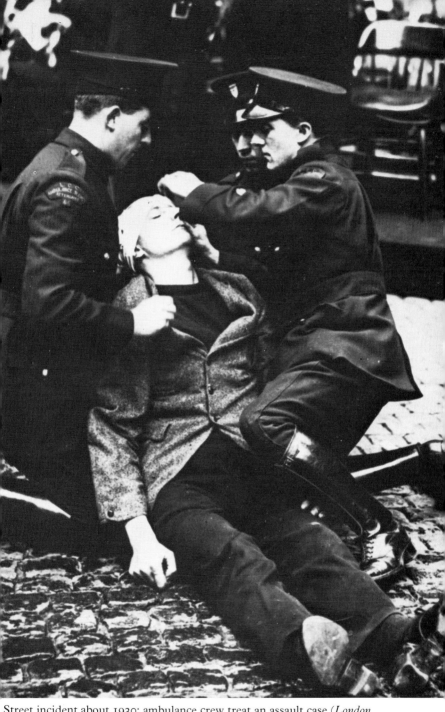

Street incident about 1930: ambulance crew treat an assault case (*London Ambulance Photo Library*)

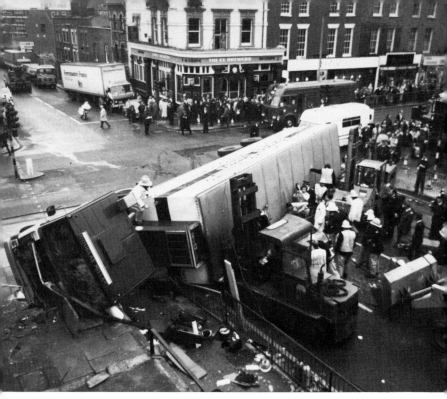

Fatal accident in London N1, 1978, when a lorry overturned at traffic lights, crushing a car

Docks worker with fractured leg is treated for severe pain (*London Ambulance Photo Library*)

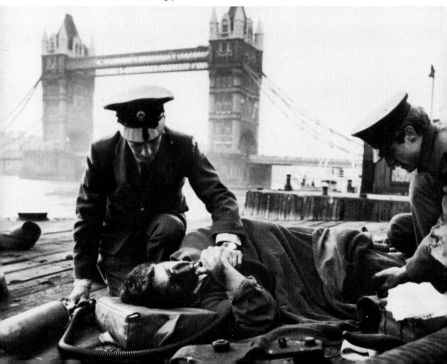

nearly as good as his!' Mick glanced at the card-player's partner, still sitting silently beside him. Then his face drained, causing Mary to rush forward, only to stop in her tracks. She too saw what was going on. 'Oh God,' she said, disgusted. Before them sat the lifeless bodies of two former patients. Their expressionless faces stared into space, their eyes wide open. One figure's mouth hung low, with his jaw nearly reaching his chest. His ashen complexion was high-lighted by a cigarette, precariously secured between his pale lips.

'Look at his luck!' the porter exclaimed and pointed at the fist of one cadaver. It clutched five cards in a rigor mortis grip, 'A Royal Flush!'

The unexpected tends to occur more frequently when a crew is forced to act on instinct and initiative, especially if it is on strange territory. This often happens when it is necessary to gain access to premises in an emergency. On one occasion a woman had made an emergency call in good faith. Her neighbour, an elderly, infirm man, had spent many years in and out of hospital, mainly with diabetic complications. One morning the woman heard his dog barking violently but could get no reply from his front door. She had also tried to contact him by telephone with no success.

The ambulance team managed to get to the call in three minutes, the case being passed to them as 'Query collapse behind locked doors'. The attending crew was fairly new, neither of them long out of Training School. Tim, attendant of the day, grabbed his immediate kit and hurried towards the anxious neighbour who was standing in the next-door garden. Mike parked the ambulance, and the neighbour, explaining why she was concerned, followed him as he went around the ground floor. He peered through all the windows, shouting the occupant's name; there was no response, nor were there any doors or windows open. 'Looks like we'll need police authorisation to break in. Perhaps he's collapsed in the bath,' suggested Mike.

'He's not too good on his feet,' the neighbour told them. 'He can walk, but he's just had an operation on his left leg.'

Tim became a little concerned. He thought about an old man lying helpless, perhaps on the verge of cardiac arrest, maybe even already unconscious. 'What do you want to do?' said Mike, urging his colleague to make a quick decision. 'Let's get the police down to break in.'

Mike hurried back to the vehicle, broke the air space and requested immediate police attendance. Red Base had, however, anticipated the problem, requesting police assistance from Scotland Yard. Tim continued to examine the house, even considering entering through a top bedroom window that appeared not quite shut. But then, just as Mike returned, Tim spotted something. As he strained his sight into a darkened rear room, he saw what looked like a shoed foot. The more he squinted into the gloomy interior, the more convinced he became. 'Mike, look behind the bed, it looks like Mr Milford.' His partner scrutinised the limb and agreed. 'That's him all right; you can see his foot clearly, but we'll have to wait for the police.'

The neighbour began to fret; Mike looked at his colleague. It was a unanimous decision: they would break in immediately.

Mike went to get the ambulance crowbar; Tim took off his jacket and placed it against one of the windows. He grabbed the iron rod from his colleague and, warning the woman to stand clear, shattered the pane, scattering tiny pieces on the dark carpet inside. The dog began to bark noisily as Tim fumbled for the inside catch and tugged hard at the window frame. They scrambled into the darkened room, Tim gripping his satchel, to be greeted by the dog, which fiercely voiced its disapproval of the trespassers. The two were forced to stand back, staring in frustration at the limp-looking foot behind the bed. Mike had an idea, however. He asked Tim to pass him a blanket that lay folded near the window. Opening the heavy material wide, he heaved it over the dog, and they were able to carry it into an adjoining room. Tim raced back to the foot of the bed but felt perplexed; still only one limb was visible. 'The man must be underneath the bed,' he concluded aloud and reached for the protruding leg. To his horror it came away in his hands. A split second later he realised what he was holding.

A man peered through the window. 'What's going on?' he demanded. Mike stood speechless. 'I see you've found my spare leg,' declared the man, who was obviously an amputee and the occupant of the house they had broken into. Tim squirmed and looked sheepishly at his colleague; Mike offered a bleak smile.

'Looks like we haven't got a leg to stand on.'

Even having been admitted to a house in the normal way, it is possible to be surprised. Once inside it is generally easy to guess income, tastes, nationality and even character, but such guesses are not always right.

One crew had the task of taking a geriatric patient to hospital. The house where the old lady lived looked as if it had not been decorated since World War I, and from the outside, compared with the rest of the street, gave the impression of being uninhabited. Grass and weeds covered the garden, and the paintwork was chipped and blistered.

Yet, as the crew removed the 70-year-old woman into the carrying chair, she clutched at her bed as if reluctant to part with it. The district nurse who was present wondered if her purse was under her pillow, but nothing was to be found; the incoherent patient, a little eccentric, continued to make a fuss. It was only when the mattress was lifted that the truth was discovered. Under her bedding, tucked up warmly and securely in a long row, lay a collection of bank-notes, packed tightly in thick wads. It transpired that there was £26,000 in all, collected over the years. Alas, the owner was now past enjoying her riches.

I also came across a family who were apparently in a position to afford expensive items, yet were quite content to live in circumstances that can only be described as disgusting. The case was passed to Greenford as 'abdominal pain, no doctor available'. As attendant that day, I made the initial contact with the family calling for help. A well-dressed man greeted me at the door, gestured towards the front room, said 'She's in there mate,' and then shouted out aloud: 'Right, I'm off to work, Joan, see you later. If you want a lift back from the hospital, phone me.' With that, he strolled down the path through a garden that would have made Percy Thrower weep and drove off in a one-year-old Italian saloon car.

As I entered the house a foul stench hit me. I coughed a few times but tried to be diplomatic. Venturing through the open doorway, the first thing I saw was what appeared to be a brand-new colour television in the far corner of the room. Though the sound was turned down, four young children sat around it as though hypnotised. The children wore similar outfits, all of which bore large holes and stains. They were not wearing shoes, and the soles of their feet were jet black.

The room itself was cluttered with all things imaginable, from old hamster cages to parts of motorbikes. Around and between most objects were strips of newspaper, which blended with the half-removed lengths of old, brown-ringed, parchment-like wallpaper. Cigarette ends littered the black carpet, yet I was only guessing that the damp furry substance underfoot was, in fact, a carpet. The coal fire in the grate burned steadily, and I could feel my cheeks becoming red. My colleague entered the room, but, seeing I was still making an evaluation, left discreetly. I understood why; I, too, was feeling a little sick.

I looked towards the sofa and heard a low moan coming from under a soiled sheet which appeared to be covering a large bag of clothes. From beneath the linen appeared the head of a middle-aged woman. She pulled back the covers, revealing an unwholesome appearance. 'I've got this pain,' she grunted. 'Come on all of a sudden.'

By now I was feeling most uncomfortable and clenched my teeth. Before I could reply I heard a rustle coming from near the window. Craning my neck, I saw some newspaper moving around in an old grocery box. From under the cover of this paper popped the head of a kitten. It scampered forward and introduced several other brothers and sisters, who were crammed together in foul conditions. I reverted my attention to my 'patient', and she continued her story. Finding that I could not stand the idea of staying in that room any longer, I offered her conveyance to the nearest hospital. I felt sure her pains were exaggerated but gave her the benefit of the doubt by offering her a carrying chair. She willingly accepted the idea, and I popped out into the welcoming fresh air to ask my partner to bring one in.

No sooner had I returned to the porch, than the lady sprang to her feet and put on a fur coat and high-heel shoes. She brushed her hair vigorously in the mirror above the fire and met me in the hallway. Behind her in the kitchen a lean greyhound stood quiet, without a whimper. Around him were stacked plates, cutlery, milk bottles and dishcloths in a disorganised, soiled array. The kitchen floor was covered with litter, including squashed milk cartons and cigarette papers.

The woman bade her children farewell, but not one of them turned a head away from the television screen. Once we had lifted the patient inside the vehicle and fastened the doors I sat opposite her, placing a blanket around her legs to keep her warm as was customary procedure. But to my surprise she discarded the blanket, pushing it to one side as if deeply offended. 'I won't if you don't mind,' she said. 'I can't be sure you haven't used that on someone else!'

Ambulance crews have sometimes been positively alarmed by the sights that greet them. Responding to a call in north London, an ambulance crew stepped into a snake-pit—quite unknowingly. The occupant of a luxury flat, obviously a lover of reptiles, beckoned them inside without warning. Before their gaze crawled snakes of every description, on the bookshelves, between newspapers, along walls and beside the sofa. In one corner, under a rubber plant, was coiled an enormous python, sleeping contentedly as if recently fed.

As well as unusual sights, unusual characters occasionally appear at the other end of an emergency call. I remember taking a call one morning at Greenford Ambulance Station. Red Base Control Officers are well known for their sense of humour, and I recorded the details given me with some scepticism: 'A speared Zulu'. I laughed at the Controller, assuming my leg was being pulled. 'What is it really?' I wanted to know.

'Just that old boy. I'll leave it with you!'

The address given was in a residential estate in Perivale, and it took four minutes to get there along Western Avenue. As we drove, Jim Lock, my present colleague, kept asking me about the call as if I had instigated it. I told him I was as confused as he was and that I presumed someone called Mr or Mrs Zulu had cut themselves. As I stood at the door of the house in Bilton Road, waiting for someone to answer the door, I could see someone wearing an enormous head-dress approaching the glass door. I smirked to myself, thinking how much it did look like a Zulu but that it must be a woman with a towel around her hair. However, as the door swung open, to my amazement it was indeed a 'Zulu'. He clutched his side and looked in pain.

'Am—Ambulance Service,' I stammered.

'Yes, won't you come inside?' the Zulu replied, in an Oxbridge accent. 'Damn silly really, I slipped on a cake of soap or something while getting out of the bath. Knocked my side against a protruding towel-rack, and I appear to be speared, as it were.' I forgot myself for a moment, studying the man's outfit with absolute amazement. He smiled. 'Are you going to do something for me?'

Apologising, I got to work, and he explained that he worked at an African Embassy and had to appear this morning in national dress for a diplomatic function. He had not lived in the house very long and had had to summon help from his unknown next-door neighbour, who had actually made the 999 call. 'He had a similar expression to yours,' the well-mannered man mused, as, still a little taken aback, I attended to his wound. Jim soon appeared in the doorway. I only wish I had had a camera to record the look on his face!

During the short period I worked in the Central London area, I was sent to many unusual locations on 999 calls—unusual for me, at least, but quite common for ambulance work in that area. The calls came from embassies, Buckingham Palace and the Houses of Parliament down to subways, overnight charity hostels and public lavatories.

At 21.50 hours one night I was on 'middle' shift at Smithfield with my temporary colleague, Tina Stovell, a pleasant, cheerful girl, aged about twenty-eight. (I never did have the courage to ask her exact age.) We had just dealt with a case of infectious meningitis and were returning from headquarters after disinfecting the vehicle and equipment. Before obtaining a 'Return to base', a further call came through on Channel 1. Tina, as attendant, responded, glancing at her wrist watch as she did so.

'Roger Smithfield 1, I have a Call Red accident.'

'Go ahead.'

'It's to the public lavatories at Charing Cross railway station. A collapse, query the cause. 21.51 Romeo Sierra Delta, Smithfield 1 over.' Tina followed procedure and read back the call to double check all the details. As we were a stone's throw from the station and the traffic was light, I did not use the blue lights as we drove smartly to Charing Cross. As we arrived at 21.54 we were met by a police constable. Picking up her immediate-aid satchel and a hand-lamp, Tina approached the officer, who explained that the patient was in the ladies' toilets. Tina went down the narrow, damp stairway, a dank mildewy smell rising to meet her. In the dimly lit interior she made out a fairly tall, well-dressed blonde, heavily made up, slumped to one side but fully conscious. Thick black mascara had mixed with flour-like face-powder and made a thin paste around her weepy eyes. Her dress covered her knees but revealed black seamed stockings and expensive-looking high-heel shoes.

I appeared in 'no-man's land' just as Tina was carrying out her initial checks, but the patient refused to speak to her, not even replying when Tina asked permission to look through her handbag in the hope of finding a clue to a possible medical problem. A phial of tablets was eventually discovered. Tina looked closely at the label then passed it to me: it read 'Phenobarb: one thrice daily. A. Carter'. We concluded that the patient suffered with epilepsy and had just had a seizure. She would need to be watched carefully during the journey to hospital in case she had another attack, but little treatment could be offered, even in a hospital casualty unit. I brought down our chair and the pre-heated shock blanket to wrap her in. We secured her to the metal-and-canvas framework of the carrying unit and managed, with only a little difficulty, to negotiate the narrow staircase.

At St Thomas' Hospital, just opposite the Houses of Parliament, the night-shift casualty staff were having a fairly quiet time for a change. We wheeled our patient in and Tina gave details to the sister on duty, who glanced at the woman and asked us to put her in a cubicle. Soon, therefore, at 22.21, we were available for further calls, and, although our duty period was due to end at 23.00 hours, we received yet another call, to a foot injury, along the Albert Embankment. At 22.44, we were back in St Thomas', this time with a young teenager who bore the signs of a possible fractured ankle, his left foot now enclosed comfortably by our air splint. The duty sister directed us to take him to another cubicle and, with a grin, asked us not to make this sort of frequent attendance a habit.

Before we could leave, the nursing sister beckoned to us. 'Would you like to see how your lady is getting on?' she asked. I realised that she was referring to our last case and nodded. 'Take a look for yourselves!'

We made our way to the cubicle in which we had left her and quickly came out. The sister nodded at us, smiling broadly. We looked again. There, lying back on the couch in the small room, was a young man of about twenty-four with crew-cut hair; beside him lay his stockings, dress, handbag, high heels and wig.

The white vehicle I drive from time to time, with its emergency lights, red-and-blue stripes and two-tone horns is on the whole regarded with reserve and a degree of respect by the public—essential if ambulance staff are to carry out their duties effectively—and on almost every occasion that an ambulance is left unattended it is unharmed. On the rare occasions when this is not the case, however, the consequences can be disastrous.

I am thinking of two or three recent instances when ambulances have been stolen. Presumably the individuals responsible wanted to live out boyhood ambitions and fantasies. Often the police eventually find the stolen vehicle a few miles away, the medical apparatus intact. Once, however, a stolen ambulance was used in a bank raid and proved to be an ideal get-away vehicle. The thieves went further, stealing or obtaining the correct uniforms, and actually having the nerve to fill up the vehicle with petrol from an accident ambulance station on their 100-mile journey to the Midlands.

Recently a crew attending a 999 call in the early morning had hurried into the house to give immediate treatment to a young boy who was having difficulty breathing during an asthma attack; when they emerged from the house, carrying the child who was in acute respiratory distress, the ambulance had vanished. It had been stolen, a callous and stupid act. The crew had to make a further 999 call and wait for another five minutes for a second emergency ambulance. Fortunately the boy recovered, although he could easily have been endangered by the delay.

One north London crew really came across the unexpected on a call. A frail lady, about to pay in some money fainted in the queue in a local high-street bank. The warm weather must have proved too much for her. The ambulance crew who attended the case, Sam and Ken, were 'old hands' with thirty-five years' experience between them; they had come across just about every possible type of situation. Sam walked into the bank first and smiled at the old lady who sat upright on a chair being looked after by a counter clerk. 'What's happened to you, eh?' he asked, sympathetically.

'I'm not too sure,' the lady replied. 'I just came over dizzy.'

'You'll have to take more water with it.' Ken breezed in and knelt by his partner. 'So this is the lady causing all the trouble,' he remarked, and was about to get up to fetch some equipment when there was a sudden flurry of activity at the doorway followed by a scream. Four armed and masked men hurled themselves into the bank. 'Anyone who gets heroic gets blasted,' threatened the biggest man of the group, scanning the frightened faces of the customers through the peep-holes in his balaclava. While his colleagues set to work, the look-out caught sight of the two ambulancemen, who in their blue uniforms resembled police officers. There was a tense moment when it seemed he was not sure. 'Hope I won't have to give you two guys any more work,' he barked, clutching his sawn-off shotgun. He had realised who they were.

Sam and Ken remained still and helpless. Sam glanced at the old lady and moved forward to hold her trembling hand. He squeezed the gloved fingers reassuringly as he watched what was going on. The thieves spent only four minutes in the bank and left as abruptly as they entered. Ken jumped to his feet and gingerly opened the door. He could see the gunmen bundle themselves and their takings into a Rover 3.5. Dashing into the street he leapt into the cab of the ambulance and called up 'priority'. He relayed the registration number of the dark blue get-away car to Red Base, which in turn informed Scotland Yard. Two squad cars, which were only minutes away, were given the information, and soon one raced past the bank, while the second screeched to a halt outside. By now the ambulance crew had several shocked people to attend to as well as their original patient. 'They never told us about this sort of thing at the interview!' mused Ken, still trembling slightly.

The police were able to catch the raiders, largely because of Ken's prompt action, but the crew agreed that they would rather stick to ambulance work than become deputies for the police.

The word 'collapse' in emergency work can have a multitude of meanings, indicating anything from severe migraine to a fatal heart attack. Unfortunately, because of the limited information given by callers, control officers have to pass on this vague statement to responding crews. One collapse call I shall never forget occurred early one wintry November morning. I was working on a night shift; my temporary partner was on overtime.

At 06.10 the red emergency phone in the Greenford watchroom shattered the peace within. I started at the sudden clatter and answered the line. It was a collapse call. I expected the worst, for most collapse cases at that time of morning are patients who have died in the night and are beyond all emergency treatment. Colin started up Greenford 1's engine, while I grabbed my jacket and scurried out into the garage, locking the swing-doors behind me. The call had come from Sudbury Hill, and as the vehicle speeded up at the junction of

Rockware Avenue, I looked about for my essential re-suscitation apparatus and climbed into the back of the ambulance, clinging to the luggage-rack with one hand and pulling the suction unit from its wall mounting. Clutching the aspirator tightly, I returned to my seat as the vehicle swung around a corner. 'You're not much of an optimist!' Colin commented, adjusting his glasses.

'I hope I'm wrong,' I replied and started to remove other items from the attendant's immediate-aid kit, which is kept within easy reach in the cab. As we drew near to the house I could see a woman wearing a light yellow dressing-gown and slippers. She waved frantically. My blood turned cold, for these were the signs of something serious, and I swung open the attendant's door, waiting for the vehicle to slow down before I could jump to the pavement. Clutching my gear, I hurried towards the white-faced elderly lady.

'Inside! Quick!' she shouted. 'He's collapsed.' I bolted into the first room; it was empty. As I emerged I could hear the woman calling to my colleague to hurry. I rushed into the next room; that too was empty. I left my equipment in the hall and called to the woman: 'Where is he, dear?'

'In the kitchen!' She was running back towards the house. I went into the kitchen: there was no one to be seen. Perhaps the woman was not quite 'with it'; perhaps she was sleep-walking—stranger things have been known. She appeared at the door. 'Is he gone?' she asked in a sorrowful voice.

'Who dear? Is who gone?'

'Joe. Has he passed away?'

I was not quite sure what to say, as Colin appeared at the door with a chair and some blankets. 'He's behind the fridge,' she explained. 'He must have died there early this morning.'

It occurred to me that I ought to look, however daft it seemed. She might have chopped up her husband for all I knew and left part of him there! Colin helped me pull out the refrigerator, thinking, I suspect, that I was sillier than the woman. But she was quite right. We were indeed too late. Behind the refrigerator lay Joe, his yellow feathers ruffled, his eyes staring and his protruding beak pointing upwards.

The lady's canary had certainly gone to meet its maker.

Night time happenings are often more bizarre than those of the day. The dark seems to bring more than its fair share of strange and unexpected calls.

It was 4 am. I glanced at my watch and repeated my call sign. Red Base asked me to stand by, and I replaced the microphone, staring at the house in darkness. Jim Lock, my permanent colleague, and I had found ourselves at a house near Allenby Road, Southall. There was no reply and no glimmer of light visible, and we could only assume that Control had been given the wrong location by the caller. My emergency call sheet read: 'Man having heart attack' and below in the remarks section 'Wife in panic'.

Jim flopped forward on to the steering-wheel; I rubbed my eyes. Neither of us was keen on night duty and sitting outside someone's lifeless home at 4 am was not our idea of fun. We had been away from the warm station since 1.30 and we longed to get back for some refreshment. 'Greenford 1 over.' Red Base came through loudly, and I asked for their message. 'Roger, Greenford. We've just been on to the wife. She assures us her husband has collapsed in bed with a heart attack.' I was just about to argue when Jim caught a glimpse of a movement at a bedroom window. I asked Control to stand by. 'There! Did you see?' Jim pointed at the window.

I could just make out someone staring at us from a first-floor window, so I got out of the cab and wandered up the path to the front-door. Before I could knock again, I saw torch light on the staircase. Jim came up behind me with a hand-lamp.

'Perhaps the fuses have gone,' suggested Jim, shining the lamp around the porch. Eventually, after more peering from behind net curtains, the front-door was inched open to reveal a middle-aged lady wearing a white nightdress.

'Yes?' she asked.

'You called for an ambulance?'

'Oh, yes.' She opened the door wide and turned the hall lights on. 'Upstairs; he's had a heart attack you know.' Jim and I rushed up the stairs, and I fumbled in the dark for the landing switch, eventually using the pen-torch that I keep in my jacket pocket. 'Back room' came the voice of the lady from behind. I opened the door and reached for the light-switch, but nothing happened.

'You'll have to use the bedside light,' instructed the woman, who had joined us on the landing. Pointing my light towards the bed, I could see the shape of a man under the bed clothes. I turned on the bedside extension lamp but before I could touch the man in the bed, he stirred and then sat up with a start.

'What's the problem?' I enquired, looking into his sleepy but normal-looking face.

'I may ask you the same question. Who on earth are you, and what are you doing here?' He squinted at the insignia of my uniform jacket. I looked at his wife, who sheepishly popped her head around the door. The man slapped his hands against his face and bleated 'Why Stella, why?' Jim and I stood back mystified. 'Last week it was the police, the week before six burly firemen and now you've called the Ambulance Service. Why?' The timid lady disappeared as the rudely awoken man reached for his spectacles. He apologised profusely for the trouble and politely saw us out of the house.

I completed my paperwork in the cab and saw the lights of the disturbed household going out. As Jim pulled away I caught sight of the woman peering again out of the window. I turned to my partner. 'I wonder who her guests will be next week?'

6

Ambulancewoman

Equal rights, pay and conditions for both sexes have been granted in ambulance work for a long while, and women have always been actively employed to carry out the complete range of ambulance duties. I have met many lady war veterans who could tell me of night time duties in the blitz, conveying patients who had been caught by an air raid. But despite their theoretic equality in the Service, many women have been aware of animosity and ill-feelings in their working environment, of negative attitudes that have been shown not only by patients but by members of allied professions and their own male colleagues. Most of the ambulancewomen with whom I have worked have been more than my equals, and their approach, training and attitudes to ambulance duties are the same as those of the men.

To the four ambulancewomen involved in the cases I describe in this chapter, I offer my greatest respect and admiration. Each of them met adversity in accepting a job that some would assume was a man's task. They have had to prove themselves under difficult and trying conditions, sometimes having to achieve far more than a man in similar circumstances.

Jean McGee, twenty-five years old and married, joined the Ambulance Service in 1977, after what she described as a humdrum job in telephone sales. She had seen a female crew manning an accident ambulance, and at about the same time saw an ambulance recruitment advertisement in a national newspaper. She applied, but was at first unsuccessful because of lack of driving experience. On the second attempt she was accepted as a trainee. She was over the moon.

During her training Jean soon realised that she was not

only in a ready-made minority group, but also the youngest on the course. It was going to be tough going. Jean recalls her first morning at Waterloo Training School. As she meekly poked her head around the door of the great hall, a sea of faces scrutinised the recruit. Jean felt a little embarrassed, almost as if she should not be there. There were other women in the group, but in the ratio of 1:5.

Jean made sure she was regarded as an equal, never shirking her duties and new responsibilities. In practice sessions, she would be willing to lift heavy 'patients' with the same enthusiasm as some of her more muscular colleagues. She did not flinch at the idea of being lowered from the side of a warehouse during rescue training, dangling in mid-air 30–40 feet up. She was determined to take it all in her stride, a determination recognised and noted by instructors, who were pleased with her attitude and progress. She was going to make the grade.

Early on during operational training, Jean McGee and her colleague, a young ex-bus driver, were called to Oxford Circus. They had 'one under' and were both nervous of what they might encounter. Jean was attendant that day and had to take the lead, making the decisions as necessary. At the underground station a police sergeant met the rescue party. He must have realised that they were only 'rookies' and smiled reassuringly at them. Jean was given a full outline of the problem: the patient was alive and on the rail. The sergeant could not help asking if the crew was up to it. 'Have you done one of these before, love?'

'No, I'm afraid it's my first.'

'Shall I ask for another crew? No one here will blame you if you just want to walk away. Not another word would be said.' It was this sort of statement that brought out Jean's feminist pride. The police officer may have been thinking only of her inexperience, but subconsciously perhaps her sex may have been the issue. 'No, please don't worry. We're more than ready to deal.' Jean turned to her colleague. 'Aren't we?' She hopped down on to the rails and dealt with her patient, oblivious of self-concern. Perhaps being under close surveillance from so many men had a lot to do with it.

When she had completed her training, Jean was posted to Hanwell Station in west London, an ambulance centre that already had quite a few women on its staff. This made her reception friendlier than she had expected, and she fitted in quickly. One job in particular will always stick in her mind: a job that was successfully dealt with only because she was a woman; one that, had she not been on duty, would have been an enormous problem to the Service.

It was a busy morning, and a male crew was called to a house just off Greenford Road. The reception the men got at the doorstep through the letterbox was not friendly. The woman inside, who refused the crew entry, was clearly in distress; her clothes, seen through the letterbox, were red with blood, and she seemed near to total collapse. The crew tried to reason with her, but all they could get was her reluctance to see men. A woman? Perhaps. The Hanwell crew contacted Red Base to ask for an ambulancewoman. Control obliged, and Jean was despatched as soon as she returned from one of her own cases.

When a woman's voice was heard at the front door, a little girl, seven or eight years old, cautiously opened up. Her frightened face alarmed Jean. What on earth was going on? 'I don't want any men. If it's a man, tell him to get out!' screamed the mother from inside the house. Jean smiled at the tearful child and walked into the rear living-room of the untidy house. What met her eyes was like a scene from *The Texas Chain-Saw Massacre*. A woman in her thirties lay on a black plastic sofa. From the sofa dripped blood which had formed a pool on the carpet. There was blood everywhere, on the curtains, carpets, tabletops and chairs. The room resembled an abbatoir. The patient stared at the ambulancewoman as if hypnotised. Her deathly pale face underlined the severity of the haemorrhage. Towels were wrapped haphazardly about her middle, pulled together tightly by blood-stained fingers. A stab wound would have been a fair assumption, but intuitively Jean knew that this was a female problem, which explained the patient's reluctance to deal with a man. 'What have you been doing?' Jean asked.

'Oh, just a heavy period.'

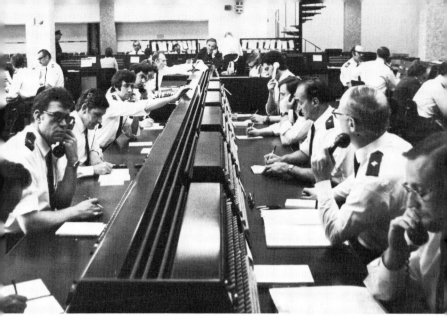

Red Base Control, nerve centre of London's ambulance service (*London Ambulance Photo Library*)

New recruits learn light rescue techniques (*London Ambulance Photo Library*)

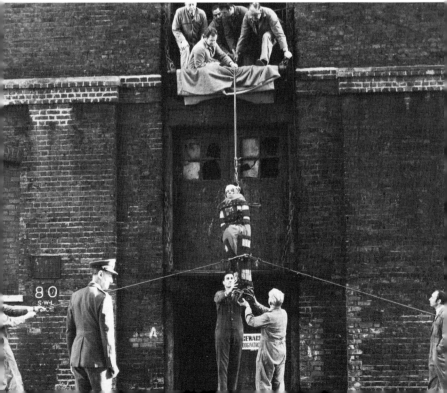

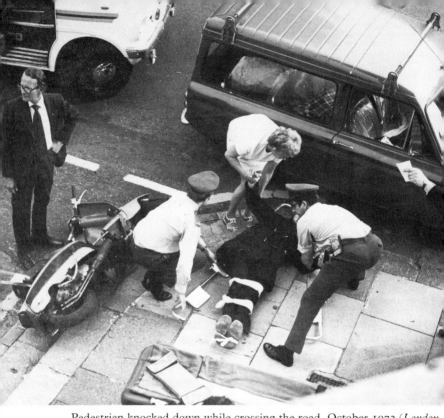

Pedestrian knocked down while crossing the road, October 1973 (*London Ambulance Photo Library*)

Bringing out a survivor on oxygen and drip during the Moorgate Underground disaster of February 1975 (*Daily Mirror*)

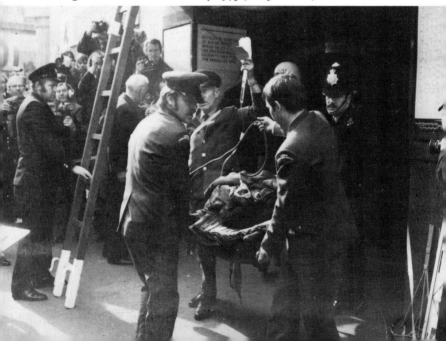

If the situation had not been so serious, Jean would have laughed aloud: 'Come on, love, do you think I'm a fool? This is no period is it? What's going on?'

The woman moved to one side as more blood oozed along her legs. 'I had to—it was the only way,' she said at last. Jean edged nearer, taking care not to slip on the red mire underfoot. 'What did you need to do? Come on, I want to help you. Let me see under the towel.' The woman pulled herself back and shouted, 'No, don't touch me.'

Jean hesitated for a moment but guessed that the woman was too weak to make much more fuss. 'Come on, you're in a terrible state, I only want to help.' Now within reaching distance, Jean stretched out to the saturated towels and pulled them away. By now a neighbour had arrived and was asked to assist. 'Get me some more clean towels and hot water, I'm going to clean the lady up,' ordered Jean, reaching in her jacket pocket for a large dressing, which she used to staunch the stream of blood.

'Your colleagues want to know if you need any help,' the neighbour enquired. Jean spoke quickly before her patient could explode into another anti-male tirade. 'No, dear, tell them I'm OK. I don't need further assistance yet.'

The lady nodded and left the room. The little girl peeped around the door. 'Are you all right, Mum?'

'Course she is,' smiled the ambulancewoman. 'Aren't you, Mum?' The patient was unable even to nod; and instead she looked away with a confused frown. 'Mummy was screaming all night,' explained the youngster. 'All after Mummy's boyfriend had left. They had an argument.'

Jean looked hard at her patient. She had already decided what the problem was and wanted the woman to admit it herself, but she refused to communicate. Later in hospital, as the patient recovered, the full story emerged: she had taken the most dangerous and agonising step a depressed pregnant woman can take, attempting a do-it-yourself abortion with a pair of knitting needles.

Maureen Browne, a young ambulancewoman at my station, has been in the Service for over ten years. She started her

career as a 'sitting-case' driver, dealing purely with out-
patients, and took the necessary training to graduate to
accident and emergency work.

I remember discussing with her the various aspects of
women in ambulance work, and she had some interesting
views. 'You're at a disadvantage straightaway,' she told me,
'because people always expect an ambulanceman to knock at
their door or arrive at an accident. One is often greeted with
"Oh, it's a lady." I think they almost feel cheated and in that
respect you have to prove that you are capable of assessing the
patient, giving treatment and driving safely to hospital
without causing an accident on the way. After all this, people
will still comment, "Isn't she good—for a girl" or "Didn't
she drive well"—which is rather an insult, considering I've
only done my job.'

Maureen has often come across that attitude, especially
when she has been working with another woman. 'The
ambulance crew has arrived—and they're both ladies!' This
goes even further when it comes to moving a patient; men
rally round to do the lifting for the crew, which is rather like
going up to a policeman at a busy road junction and taking
over the traffic direction.

During the time Maureen worked permanently with
another woman, the crew received an accident call to the Golf
Links Estate, Southall, a large complex of flats in the Ealing
area. This case was passed to the ambulance station as
'Overdose, unconscious'. It was late evening as Greenford 3
turned into Fleming Road and made its way across the vast
council estate. After a little searching Maureen spotted the
correct block and left the ambulance while her colleague
parked. It was easy to get lost in the tower block and Maureen
waited by the lift for her partner. Together they went up to
the eighth floor to find the flat. The door was eventually
opened by a woman.

'Oh yes, he's in here,' she whispered. On the floor at the
end of the short corridor lay a well-built man, flat on his
stomach. Maureen went up to the man, turning his face to one
side to check his level of consciousness. This proved unnecessary. As soon as she touched his face, the man opened

his eyes wide, and, scrambling to his feet, he shot past her, producing as he moved a slender steel blade. Maureen's colleague stepped aside in surprise, not fully appreciating what was happening, as the man kicked the door shut. He turned to the three women. 'No one is going anywhere!' he threatened, looking at each of his captives in turn. Maureen felt her body stiffen and her heart pound. Three unarmed women against a man holding a dagger.

Maureen considered what emergency action they might take. If the worst came to worst, could they perhaps disarm the man in a unified attack? Would she have to make the first move? Was the other woman, now standing in the narrow hall, on their side?

There was silence: the man lowered the knife and slumped against the wall, perhaps considering his next move. Maureen whispered to the other woman, who turned out to be his girlfriend. She had become concerned when the man, who had been depressed, had fallen to the floor after too much drink, and she had been unable to rouse him. As Maureen listened to the story, she kept her eyes on the man who was beginning to look threatening again. Just then, as the ambulancewoman was considering extreme measures, some words of comfort came from the girlfriend: 'I've called the police as well.'

The next five minutes were tense, but then the sound of the lift was followed by heavy footsteps. Almost unbelievably, the man himself opened the front-door, only to see three uniformed policemen approaching. He bolted into the corridor and was promptly pursued by two of the officers. The third came in, to the relief of the ambulance crew and girlfriend. They heard a scuffle outside, then heard the man being arrested.

It was an experience Maureen would not wish to go through again, but at the same time she did not regard it as a case for an all-male crew. If two ambulancemen had appeared, the man might have used his knife without a second thought.

Maureen once conveyed to hospital a pop-singer who had turned to alcohol. She had to accompany him from Mount

Vernon Hospital to St Bernard's, some twelve miles away, a journey long enough for a lengthy conversation. She felt sorry for the ex-star, who had been very successful in the sixties, and she was curious to know why he had turned his back on success. In the confined space of the ambulance, he poured out his heart, but it was not until they arrived at St Bernard's that Maureen realised what complications her genuine sympathy with, and keen interest in, all the man had said, had caused. 'I've fallen in love with you,' he told her. Maureen was stunned. She did not know quite what to say. 'Will you come and visit me, please?' he implored.

'I don't know,' she replied, redfaced at the outcome of her friendly chat. For days afterwards Maureen thought about the man; perhaps a visit would cheer him up, maybe even stop his alcoholism. But then she could also be playing with his emotions and that would make matters worse. The golden rule about not getting involved with patients had to be enforced for both their sakes.

The Load of Hay is a public house in Northolt, at the junction of Eastcote Lane North. It is a busy traffic intersection that sees its fair share of road accidents. Soon after Maureen had joined the Service, she was called to the junction for a serious RTA. A policeman met her and her partner and explained that the patient was dead. There could be no doubt: his head had been crushed by the wheels of a lorry. The Fire Brigade had been summoned, and they were going to free the body by jacking up the lorry. The ambulance crew's task would be to remove the patient's remains as required by law. 'Will you two stand by?' asked the officer, turning away to direct oncoming cars.

Maureen was nervous about the work she knew she had to do, but that was not solely her concern. There was clearly going to be an all-male gathering—half a dozen policemen, her own colleague and the fire crew. She knew from previous experience that, as attendant, she would be the focus of attention when the time came for her to act, in a situation that would make most women squirm. Her concern about being seen by other male emergency workers as visibly nervous only made her more anxious. The waiting made it worse. It would be several more minutes before they could remove the unfortunate victim. Maureen kept telling herself to keep calm so that she did not show herself up and let the women's side down. Then something happened that saved the day.

A young police constable came up to the ambulance crew, his notebook in his hands, to get some information about the ambulance call. 'Got your times, love?' he asked. Maureen reached for the clipboard and read off the relevant information. She noticed the constable's hands, which shook so much that what he wrote was almost indecipherable. He too found the incident distressing. This was a wonderfully reassuring sight to her: she was nervous no more!

I first met Jean Richardson when she came to Hanwell Ambulance Station in 1975. A lively, intelligent girl, she had a smile that won her a lot of friends as well as cheering up many a forlorn patient. When my partner left the Service around this time, Jean was assigned to work with me at Greenford. I had no qualms about working with a woman and saw her greater professional experience as a way to increase my own abilities, which proved to be the case. Over the couple of years I had the pleasure of working with her, she passed on a wealth of knowledge.

She had joined the Ambulance Service after seeing many of her friends do the same. They would talk at length about the satisfaction and interest the work offered, an exciting career that was also worthwhile. Yet it was not until Jean was involved in a road accident that she decided to take the plunge herself. She remembers a dark country lane and a motorcyclist somersaulting over a car's bonnet. Jean was the only one conscious, and was at a loss to know what to do; she felt useless, desperately wishing she at least had some first-aid training. She subsequently successfully applied to the London Ambulance Service.

During her spell in the Training School she found it necessary to assert herself. She recalls being one of three women on the course and feeling left out when it came to crewing up for duties; the men were reluctant to have a woman as a partner. It was a trying time, and it was only after a call to Leicester Square that she finally felt accepted. Called to a drug overdose in the men's lavatories, Jean's training officer expected female reserve to come into play, but this was not the case. Jean knew she had a job to do and wasted no time feeling embarrassed or out of place. She dismissed social niceties and went straight into the male preserve to commence work on her casualty. This impressed her supervisor, and from that moment on she was looked upon with much respect.

Having completed her time at Waterloo, Jean was posted to Isleworth, where she eventually crewed up with another woman. This happened more by chance than by design, and it was a bit of a novelty to be part of the only all-female crew at the ambulance station. However, they still had to prove themselves.

An accident hear Hampton Court had trapped several people in a car. When Jean and her colleague Mal arrived, there was organised chaos; the Police and Fire Brigade had surrounded the wrecked vehicle and were attempting to extract casualties. Mal and Jean parked as near to the incident as possible and threaded their way to the car through the lines of fire engines and police cars. Jean politely patted the shoulder of a uniformed policeman who had his head halfway into the vehicle. He turned, seemed to look through her and resumed his task of trying to remove a woman from the back seat. This infuriated Mal, a well-built woman, and she leaned forward and tried the officer again. 'For God's sake, let us check these patients before you move them and do untold damage!'

Again the crew was ignored. Impulsively, Mal gripped her immediate-aid satchel and slammed it hard against the constable's back. This had the desired effect, and he turned about sharply on the spot, glaring at the resolute ambulancewoman. 'What the hell are you doing?'

'Ambulance Service,' replied Jean angrily, pointing to her shoulder flash. Reluctantly the officer stepped aside and allowed the ambulancewomen to take over—but what a performance they had to go through! The policeman later admitted that he had not recognised them as an ambulance crew, particularly as they were two ladies.

Once, when Jean was working with Maureen, they were called to a golf club in the Ealing area in response to a heart-attack call. Their prompt arrival caused a problem. The steward who met them at the door looked at them blankly. 'Oh, two ladies?'

'That's right.'

'Er, well, you'll have to go round.'

'Why? Where's the patient?'

'Through this door, but you'll have to go round, you can't come in here.'

'Whyever not?'

'Well, this is the men's changing room.'

'Don't be daft, let us in.'

'Sorry, club rules, no ladies allowed.'

Jean and Maureen looked at each other in amazement. They could not believe that a heart-attack case was being kept waiting just because they were women. Eventually, after further ridiculous statements from the steward, he agreed to a compromise. 'Just wait here,' he instructed. He went into the changing room and announced: 'Gentlemen, your attention please. In a few moments two ladies will be walking through here. Thank you.' Returning to the crew, he invited them to enter. 'Promise we'll look straight ahead,' said Maureen jokingly. 'Thank you, I would be obliged,' replied the steward entirely seriously.

Perhaps the sport itself had something to do with the ambulancewomen's embarrassed reception. If they have had to attend an injured player in a football team's changing room, no announcement is made, though towels are grabbed left, right and centre. Instead of reluctance, they hear such cheery chat as: 'You can examine *me*, love,' and 'I've got this pain in my back.'

The members of an all-woman crew have to face exactly the same problems as two men. They must deal with violent mental patients as well as Saturday night drunks. Only rarely do they call for assistance, and then for the police to make an arrest. One ambulancewoman was stabbed with her own pair of scissors by a psychotic patient—fortunately not seriously; she received no more sympathy from the Service than an ambulanceman would.

One night, at 23.41, when Jean was working with an ambulancewoman who is no longer in the Service, they were called to a location near a public house, which lay back from the main road. The two street lamps in front of the pub were defective, and the area was dark. The patient, a man who had been seriously assaulted, was lying in the middle of the road. Jean turned on her auxiliary fog-lamps as she pulled up in front of the man. There were no police about, nor any bystanders. Jean's partner leapt out of the cab with a hand-lamp, medical kit and blanket, while Jean switched on the hazard-warning lights to supplement the blue beacons and give warning to other traffic.

It was only when the ambulance attendant reached the casualty that her attention was briefly drawn to the public-house car park where she could make out several shapes standing around motorbikes. The young victim, who lay face down, was unconscious, with a bleeding head wound. Suddenly, the shapes in the car park attacked another man, and Jean raced to the cab to call for immediate police assistance. As she called through to Control, a group of young tearaways stormed out across the ambulance headlights like a stamped-ing herd of cattle. Fighting broke out between two rival gangs, but no one took any interest in the ambulance crew as they tended the seriously assaulted patient. The police eventually arrived and sorted out the scuffle—but not before time.

If there was one thing Cindy Paddam could not stand it was accidents involving children. She vividly remembers a 'cot death' when the mother of the child was so shocked that she became a zombie, walking around her own home in a daze; while Cindy's colleague tried to deal with her, she decided to blanket the lifeless outline of the infant, and with great care carried the tiny shape downstairs. It was only after a few moments that she realised what she was doing: there, at the bottom of the staircase, she stood rocking the baby—by pure force of habit and maternal instinct. Bereavement and tragedy are a part of the job. Cindy once attended two fatal road accidents, one after the other, both involving three-year-old children. Never before had she felt so bitter about life.

Now in her thirties, Cindy has been in the Service for ten years, during which time she has seen life as few women ever get to see it. Many of her experiences have been bizarre, and these have often occurred in close succession. During one night shift she received four calls: (1) male shot in face with buckshot rifle; still conscious but face cut and blasted beyond reasonable recognition. Possible gangland reprisal. (2) Two men shot with sawn-off shotgun in White Hart public house. One patient with severe injury to leg, other uninjured—bullet ricocheted off metal darts-case carried in top pocket. (3) Suicide attempt; victim with one foot in a bowl of water, the other connected to household mains supply. (4) Successful suicide: using household flex, man hung himself from top stairwell in block of flats. Rarely, fortunately, do crews receive such a horrific list of calls all in the same shift, but it does happen.

Rather like the rest of her lady colleagues, Cindy had a tough time proving she was more than a pretty hairdo and a neat set of manicured fingernails. Her first-ever partner so detested the idea of working with a woman that he refused to speak to her for two weeks! Ambulancewomen are occasionally compared with nurses, but tough as their jobs may be, nurses rarely have to risk life and limb to get to a patient; they hardly ever find accident victims under rubble or on top of warehouse buildings.

Cindy was recently called to a sports field where a pavilion was being demolished. A workman had been injured; few details about his condition were given to Red Base, just that he had fallen. A plump Irishman met the crew and explained that the injured man was up on the roof. Apparently he had been blown off by a gust of wind and had landed in the rafters; this was fortunate for him as there was not much of the building left, and below him was a long drop to the ground.

Cindy loathed heights, but said nothing to her partner, Danny, who was manoeuvring the ambulance. She pressed on alone to the top of the partly destroyed pavilion, where she got a shock. The route to her casualty was a catwalk no more than twelve inches wide. 'My God,' she gasped under her breath, staring at the emptiness beneath. 'Take my hand, lovey,' offered the workman, but Cindy had other ideas. If this rather well-built man were to slip and fall, she would surely go with him. 'No, thanks all the same; I'll manage.' It was going to be the longest thirty feet Cindy had ever walked. It was only concern for her patient that had got her this far. 'Don't look down,' barked the Irishman, but it was easier said than done. One false move on the wet board would surely mean an early retirement.

Stepping out gingerly, she trekked across the narrow plank as if performing a high-wire act. To say that she was frightened would be an understatement, but she eventually reached her patient and was pleased, for both their sakes, that the injury was minor, a sprained ankle at worst. But how were they going to get back?

After attending to the man's foot, Cindy considered various methods of removal, all of which would be too dangerous across that catwalk. The patient suggested that he might be able to put some weight on his foot and hobbled up to give it a try. Cindy reassured her charge that all would be well, but another glance below did her no good at all. The more she convinced the man that there was nothing to worry about, the more she wished someone would give similar reassurance to her. Together, patient and rescuer inched their way back to safety in each other's arms.

After the incident, she reflected on the risk she had taken, perhaps a greater one than she had realised at the time. If a gust of wind had blown the fairly heavy man from his perch, how easy it would have been then for the same thing to have happened to her . . .

The other case that froze Cindy's blood started with a television set on the pavement outside a two-storey house. It had been thrown from an upper bedroom window, and a heap of wood and electronic components lay on the concrete pavement. This was not a good sign, and the crew went up the stairs cautiously. The door to the flat was wide open, and they crept inside to look for the occupant. In the lounge they could hear what sounded like a lion prowling to and fro. A rotund man, his beard like a mane, looked disapprovingly at the two uniformed figures.

'Would you like to come with us to hospital, sir?' Cindy tried the polite, formal approach.

The man glared at the crew again, and, before the ambulance crew could say any more he strode across the room and grabbed a fully grown cat. Before their eyes, he strangled it with his powerful hands, thrusting the lifeless creature over his shoulder. 'Touch me!' he yelled, 'and I'll do that to you!'

A diplomatic retreat was in order, and sedation had to be ordered before the disturbed man could be compulsorily admitted to a specialist hospital.

Mental upsets are responsible for many ambulance calls: the depraved and violent assault others; the senile and confused hurt themselves by accident; the mildly depressed seeking attention take token overdoses; the acutely disturbed psychotics ensure their end is swift and permanent. Cindy and a temporary mate were summoned to a collapse case. A young coloured girl answered the door. 'I think my husband's dead,' she announced in a daze and slunk back into the kitchen.

'Where is he?'

'Top landing.'

On the first floor of the terraced house a man lay face down. The ambulancewoman trudged over a soaking wet carpet and reached down to feel his pulse; she turned the patient's head. Further checks made it clear that he was dead. The circumstances seemed a little suspicious, and the crew decided to call for the police. Meanwhile, Cindy was becoming increasingly aware of a burning smell: to her astonishment, the body was smoking from mid-torso. Cindy recalled her partner to witness this strange sight, and they found that the man was wired up to the household electricity supply. An experienced electrician, he had decided to end it all by saturating the upper-hall carpet, wiring his body appropriately to the 240-volt supply and suffering the obvious consequences.

Apart from the bizarre nature of the suicide, the horror of

it all was that Cindy could also have been a victim of the electrician's folly. The corpse was most certainly 'live' and deadly when Cindy first saw it, and it was only by disturbing the circuit (a lead fell off the patient's wrist as she took his pulse) that she survived.

Finally, to end this section, I must relate what was perhaps Cindy Paddam's most extraordinary incident. It was a wintry February morning, the ground carpeted with a layer of ice and frost. Cars on their way to work during the rush hour coughed clouds of grey combustion fumes. Cindy expected a busy shift of 'falls' and traffic accidents, but her first call in the thick traffic at 08.45 was a railway incident. 'Man found on line; query knocked over by train.'

'Not a nice way to begin the day,' she remarked to her colleague, 'especially before breakfast.' The call was to Ealing Broadway Underground Station, and the crew went to an area off the platform, down the line heading out of the station. Cindy was relieved to see that the patient was in one piece. Even after careful examination it was difficult to know exactly where he was fatally injured: there was a trace of blood, a tiny spot, on his shirt, but no other marks or abnormalities were visible.

The crew lifted the dead man and placed him on a rigid stretcher supplied by the staff. Rigor mortis was in evidence, and Cindy enlisted some reluctant helpers to help remove the body to the ambulance. A police car waited outside the station amid a growing crowd of bystanders. Cindy told them that it was a fatal case, informing Red Base of the same when she got back to the ambulance. 'We'll get the patient certified, then proceed to the mortuary,' she explained to the police, who peered into the ambulance. 'Roger, meet you there.' Cindy turned to speak to her partner but before she could open her mouth a scream filled the ambulance: a station porter, who had helped move the body had leapt from his seat in panic.

'What on earth's the matter?' asked one of the police officers.

'The corpse! It moved its eyes!' He yelled and disappeared into the station. 'You imagined it,' Cindy called after him. 'Poor fellow's upset. You can't be more deceased that this poor chap.' But then Cindy got the shock of her career—the 'dead' body moved its eyes sideways. She froze: was she losing control of her senses? No; the eyes of this 'deceased' person *had* moved. Logic demanded that the 'corpse' was not a corpse. She shouted to a surprised colleague to alert the nearest casualty for a 'crash' call.

The police were also taken aback at the crew's flurry of activity but, asking no further questions, they followed the ambulance through the rush-hour streets. Two-tone horns cleared a path as the two vehicles exceeded the speed limit. Cindy had only instinct to go on; the patient had no pulse, no respiration—nothing; there was extensive rigor mortis and, to all intents and purposes, the man was dead. But his eyes had moved . . . any explanation would have to be left to people with greater medical knowledge.

Just before the ambulance turned into the hospital grounds, the man's eyes moved again. Cindy herself knew she was not dreaming, but she was going to have a tough time convincing the others. As the ambulance lurched to a stop outside accident and emergency, a male nurse and casualty doctor tumbled inside, only to see a lifeless body. 'Did you put in that crash call?' questioned the doctor irritably.

'That's correct.' Cindy stood firm.

'But this man has rigor mortis.' The physician made a swift examination. 'I'd say he's been dead for at least eight hours.'

'Well, that may be so, doctor, but I have seen his eyes move.'

'Preposterous!'

'Twice.'

'Have you been overworking? Perhaps you've been drinking on duty?'

'Doctor, please believe me. I did not imagine it. That man moved his eyes.' The male nurse stepped over to Cindy and put his hand on her shoulder. 'There, I can see you're upset. You can't save every life you know.' This made matters worse. Cindy removed his hand sharply. 'I resent your attitude. I'd ask you both to take this matter a little more seriously!' Taken aback by her determination the two men leaned forward to look at the patient's eyes in half-mocking fashion which did little for Cindy's blood pressure. She stared at the motionless body, willing it to move again. Her prayers were answered: the eyes flicked from side to side.

The casualty doctor's face dropped, and he ordered the patient to be taken to the resuscitation theatre. A second crash call went out. It seemed inexplicable, but this 'corpse' was alive. Cindy rushed the patient into the special-care room; it was one of her most baffling cases, one that would be unlikely to occur again in her career, or for that matter in the doctor's. It was finally declared a case of 'suspended animation'. Incredible as it may seem, the patient's body, except his heart and lungs, was dead. Even though there was no proper heartbeat or respiration, cardiac activity was taking place and showed up as the faintest trace on an ECG monitor.

It soon became clear what had happened. He had been drunk the night before and walked down the line from the Ealing Broadway platform. He had been hit by something or someone and had fallen unconscious on the track of the siding. The sub-zero temperature during the night reduced his body-heat to unnatural levels and prevented all normal body functions except pulmonary circulation—the heart and lungs—which continued largely because of the alcohol in the bloodstream. This kept the small circulatory path warm and moving—but only just.

In hospital, he had to be thawed out slowly. Unfortunately, his brain ceased to function further, although his heart soon resumed a more regular pattern. He continued 'alive' for another seven days but eventually succumbed to cardiac failure. Cindy always remembers the incident; indeed, it would be hard to forget. Had she backed down, the 'corpse' would have been taken to the mortuary in the first instance and, though the end result would have been the same, her conscience would have been permanently uneasy.

Cindy, and her other women colleagues, never seek special recognition for the hazardous tasks they are sometimes called upon to perform. To do so would undermine their insistence on being treated exactly as their male partners are. Fortunately however, their problems with colleagues have decreased with the passing years.

7

Developing a
Sense of Humour

My work is generally a serious business, as I am so frequently in contact with sorrow, grief, concern, alarm and anxiety, which has to be met with a cool head and an objective, professional manner. To take such experiences to heart would be an intolerable strain. Many new recruits leave the Service because they feel incapable of coping with the unpleasant emotions they have to face. In fact, I nearly left after six months. I used to take distressing cases to heart, going home to think about the unfortunate patients I had dealt with on that shift, and inevitably my family and friends were affected. I had to learn that whatever he sees and feels during his work, at the end of the day an ambulanceman has to forget them all, for his own sake and sanity.

This is perhaps the main reason for the happy, relaxed personalities that most ambulance personnel try to project to the people they meet. It undoubtedly cheers and helps patients, reassuring them at distressing times. From their earliest training, new ambulance staff come into contact with the sense of humour that the Service is famed for.

From the moment I walked into the headquarters building at Waterloo on my first day, I could sense the friendly atmosphere. Instructors punctuated training with light-hearted cracks and it was not long before I too saw the lighter side of life. One incident I shall not forget occurred after the first month in the classroom. By that time we had got to know each other quite well. There were the quiet ones, the noisy ones and the odd know-it-all. Sydney Westcott was just eighteen-and-a-half, and immature even for that age. He would often try to project an image of self-assurance and great intellect, succeeding merely in betraying himself for what he was. I could never understand how he had been accepted for ambulance work. (Happily, for his own sake and that of the general public, he failed his final assessments.)

It was 11 am. After a short coffee break, course 326 reconvened in the main lecture theatre for the next instalment of our physiology syllabus. We waited for the lecturer, the Ambulance Service Medical Officer. A large anatomical model stood in front of the seating area beside the blackboard and overhead projection unit. Michael Mayor, a complete contrast to Sydney Westcott, referred to his notes as he approached it, looking around in a friendly manner. 'Have you lot familiarised yourselves with Arthur's insides?' A handful of trainees gathered round, as Michael almost began to give the lecture himself. 'Right, name the three major sections of the colon,' he paused. 'Come on, you should all know by now.'

'OK Mick, if you're so clever.' Michael took the hint.

'Ascending, descending and transverse.' He grinned at them cheekily. I saw someone else taking an interest.

'I knew that,' said Sydney Westcott arrogantly. We all groaned. Sydney approached 'Arthur'. It was obvious Michael had had enough of Sydney's conceit, but to our surprise he suddenly took an entirely new approach.

'Yeah Sydney, I do believe you did.' Sydney looked pleased as Michael came forward and took the young trainee aside. 'Between you and me, Syd,' Michael whispered, 'I really don't know why we bother coming to these lectures. I mean we are obviously on top of our subject—agreed?' Sydney nodded, surprised at what was being said to him. 'I'm sure I could point to any part of Arthur here and you'd know what it was instantly,' Michael continued. 'Like this bit here at the base of the caecum.'

Sydney peered at the fabricated anatomical protrusion. 'That's the appendix, Mick.' He looked to Michael for praise.

'Oh Sydney, no, I can't believe it. I thought you of all people wouldn't be so layman–like about the appendix.' Sydney was taken aback. 'You mean there's another medical term for the appendix?'

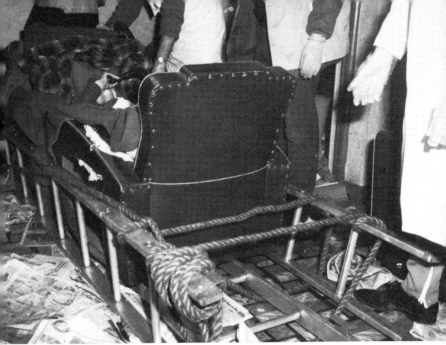

Difficult removal of an immobile elderly woman left for two months on two armchairs, October 1977

Ambulance crew rescue a trapped patient from a car involved in a head-on collision (*Clifford C. Ashton*)

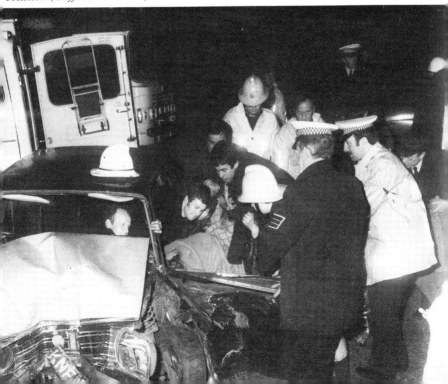

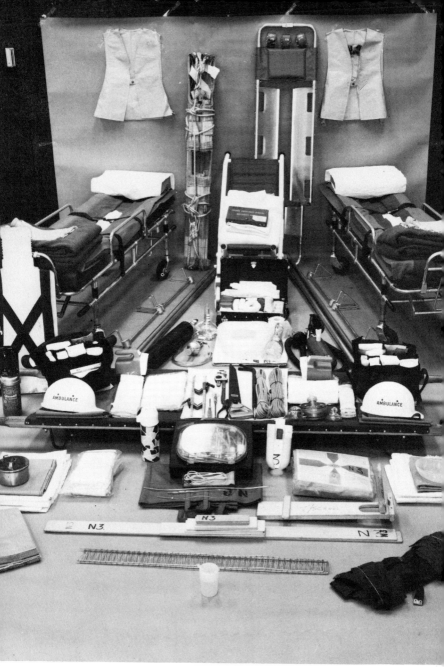

Some of the equipment carried in an accident ambulance (*London Ambulance Photo Library*)

'Of course,' insisted Michael, seriously, turning aside to wink at the rest of us. He whispered to Sydney just as the doctor entered the lecture theatre. We took our places and prepared for the lesson.

Within five minutes the discussion on the alimentary canal and human digestion was well under way, the doctor firing questions at the course. 'And now, this section of the ascending colon is the caecum as you have just told me. What is there here on the end of caecum?'

Sydney Westcott's hand shot up before anyone had even considered offering an answer. 'Yes, Mr Westcott?'

Sydney put his hand down and smiled knowingly: 'The clitoris, sir.'

I too had been the butt of much humour at training school, going out on calls with L-plates attached to my back or having the trolley-beds unfastened so that as I drove out of the garage they would roll around the back of the ambulance. It was important to accept the jokes in the spirit intended, especially when they were self-inflicted.

I remember that after a few weeks of training I suddenly became acutely aware of my new profession. I would constantly scan the horizon and my surroundings for accidents. I would look carefully at overweight men and frail old ladies, wondering if they were about to collapse in front of me so that I could leap upon them to perform my duty. Wearing a crisp new uniform made me feel ready for action should the need arise. On the second day that I was wearing that new uniform I thought my moment had come. There, on the platform of Leicester Square station, arrived a pale, breathless man, who hurried in my direction. 'This is it,' I thought. 'He's about to collapse.' My muscles tensed and I stretched out my hands to meet him, supporting him by both arms, mentally formulating my first words of reassurance; but he spoke first, withdrawing from my grasp. 'Excuse me, when's your next train for Brixton? I'm in a hurry.'

That same day, as I walked towards the ticket booth at Waterloo, a little deflated at being confused with a railway employee, my eyes fell on a 'real' patient, lying flat on his back outside the ticket office. My pulse quickened and I walked towards the ticket collector who stood, looking uninterested, near the 'casualty'. 'I'm an ambulanceman,' I said. 'May I assist?'

He glanced in my direction. 'Are you the real ambulance or are you just passing?' I reflected. It seemed a strange question. 'Well, I'm on my way to work actually.'

'Yeah, well we've called an ambulance.' He looked away to deal with a few more passengers.

'May I check him over?' I said, concerned.

The ticket collector huffed: 'If you must.'

I bent over the man, who was conscious but a little drowsy. As far as I could make out he had a slight bump on his head and, from the smell of his breath, I could guess the reason for the fall. As I examined the head injury (the first I had ever seen in my new professional capacity), I felt a hand on my shoulder. Turning, I saw one of my colleagues on the training course, also on his way to work. 'What have we got?' he chirped as if an old hand already. 'Looks like a head injury,' I told him. 'I'll check his legs,' he replied, running his trembling hands over the poorly dressed patient.

It didn't take long before we had agreed that there was no grave problem, and we merely turned the man on his side; since an ambulance was on its way, we decided to continue our journey to the Training School. After walking about fifty yards, I glanced over my shoulder. Approaching the same drunken man were two more ambulance uniforms, and the ticket collector was being badgered again. I realised why he had been so offhand: we must have been the fifth pair of trainees to offer help that morning. Waterloo was the station where most of us alighted, and a constant flow of 'freshers' would be passing through that ticket barrier. Feeling a little embarrassed I walked on, but before I turned the corner into the street, I looked back again. I could spot no fewer than four brand-new ambulance uniforms elevating the drunk's arms and legs in all directions!

I did not know what to expect after training. About ten of us were posted to the North West Division one Monday morning; my station was Park Royal, NW10. I soon found myself among a friendly bunch, who instantly made me feel at home—and became involved in some of the nonsense going on at quiet times. One established ritual for young new recruits was to be strapped into a Neil Robertson stretcher, a five-foot-long canvas device which is normally used to lower patients from tall buildings or to restrain those who need a secure bond on the way to hospital. Once the ropes and lashings are fastened, it is most unlikely that the average person will 'escape'. I was no exception, and I was tossed through the air and my head hosed down for good measure. Some unfortunate victims have been suspended six feet above ground in the garage and photographed; others have been stood upright in a bus queue of morning commuters.

Every ambulance has an isolation switch that cuts the electrical circuit of the vehicle. It is a useful anti-theft device, but it may be utilised in another way, and many is the time that I have been caught out. The isolation unit is engaged, then the two-tone horns, bell, blue lights, hazard-warning device, fog-lights, headlights, reversing lights and wind-screen wipers are switched on. The ambulance is then parked innocently on the forecourt, facing the main road. An unsuspecting recruit, as I then was, would begin a vehicle check at the start of duty and would notice that the isolation switch was down. Without another thought, he would reach down for the concealed button. As if celebrating New Year at the stroke of midnight, the quiet ambulance would spring to life, attracting the attention of everyone for miles. The recruit is then observed fumbling for switches in every direction and invariably making matters worse, cursing at having been caught out—again.

I too have caught out new faces, perhaps organising card games that have no rules, watching my pre-selected subject desperately trying to remember each move of the fictitious event. Without exception, all pranks are taken in good heart, and the working relationship among crews during their duty periods is uniformly good. The most humour, however, springs from situations that take place outside the confines of the ambulance station.

At half-past midnight a south London crew once proceeded to a call, not having been given much information. The caller had given an address and a vague message about childbirth, before mysteriously being cut off. The crew raced to the address, assuming a delivery would be necessary. Although the house was in darkness when they arrived, the attendant could see that the front door was partly ajar; indeed a mat had been placed to prevent the door from closing. His colleague went to get a torch while the attendant stood thoughtfully. It all seemed rather strange. He swung the door open and called into the darkness; there was no reply. Instead a muffled noise could be heard coming from the upper portion of the house. The crew decided to investigate. Not bothering to find the lights, the attendant led the way, using his torch to light the way. The scuffling noise increased. Opening the rear bedroom door, he shone his torch on the floor before him and saw two prostrate bodies. A young man lay over a woman, in what appeared to the ambulanceman to be a desperate effort at mouth-to-mouth resuscitation.

'I'll take over,' hollered the attendant, as the man sprang to his feet, clad only in a scanty pair of briefs.

'What the hell's going on?' (He used far stronger language.) The attendant's colleague switched on the main light, and a young woman tugged at a bedsheet in an effort to cover her almost nude body.

'Who are you? What on earth do you mean breaking into our home?'

'We got a 999 call here, something about someone having a baby.'

'What do you mean!' raved the irate lover racing about the room for something to wear. 'We only got married this afternoon.'

My initial reaction to mortuaries was one of alarm and despondency; I had always connected such places with horrific sights. I once found myself working with someone who, although much older than myself and with much more experience, shared my reservations.

One early shift we took a patient from a house in north London. He had died some time before we had been called, but for the family's sake, to alleviate their obvious distress, we had agreed to take the body to a public mortuary after the general practitioner had certified death.

I always regarded the mortuary in question with curiosity. It stood outside some park-gates that bore the helpful notice: 'No entry when gates are shut.' The building itself was behind a modern residence, and I learned that the mortician lived on the premises as part of his work, an idea that took me aback. To deliver a body we had to make an approach at the front door. On this occasion the mortician's wife answered. 'We've . . . er . . . got . . .' I did not know how to put it.

'Oh, yes,' she said, helping me out of my awkwardness. 'My husband's around the back, but you may have to wait till he comes out. I think he's got his hands full at present on a post-mortem.' I heard the news unenthusiastically and ambled to the rear of the house with my colleague, Eddie.

'God, I hate these places,' complained Eddie. 'I really don't know how people can do this type of work.' I nodded agreement as we stood outside the small building, which was at right angles to the kitchen-window of the house. Eddie was about to continue his list of grievances, but was stopped by a sudden piercing whine. It made a drilling sound as if slicing through some hard substance. 'He's going through some bones,' gulped Eddie, his face drained. 'How do you know?' I asked innocently. 'Heard it all too often mate. In a moment he'll change the tool for a saw—and you must know what that's for!'

'More bones perhaps?'

'For sawing the head off,' exclaimed Eddie, who by now did not look well. And sure enough, I could soon hear the distinct sound of a rotary blade. I felt a bit queasy as I imagined what was going on inside the mortuary. The shrill vibrations of the spinning disc met our ears. Eddie took a deep breath. 'I can even get the smell.' I sniffed and had to agree that there was an unpleasant odour in the air. The sawing continued. Then, to our horror, there was a dull thud as if a heavy weight had fallen on the concrete floor.

'He's dropped the head!' said Eddie, nauseated. 'I'm going to sit in the ambulance, I've had enough.'

Seconds later, the door swung open and a well-dressed man wearing a rubber apron and gloves emerged. The fetid odour still clung in my nostrils and I coughed. 'Hello, we've brought one for you.'

'Oh, right,' replied the mortician with a smile. 'Come in and I'll find you a space.

My stomach turned over as I reluctantly followed the man. I could not help putting my hand over my nose and mouth as I approached the doorway. 'Sorry about the smell,' he remarked. 'My wife's slung out the remains of two chickens in that bin behind you and the dustman never came yesterday.' I removed my hand, feeling foolish, and stepped inside keeping my eyes directly ahead of me.

'Over here will do.' He pointed in the direction I was trying at all costs to avoid, but I realised that sooner or later I should have to look. Turning my head slowly, I saw, in the centre of the mortician's slab, a half-constructed bedside cabinet.

'Got to do something when it gets quiet,' he commented. 'Do you like it?'

There have been times when I longed to laugh when on a call, but have had to restrain myself, unless of course the patient was laughing too. The casualty who needs emergency help for injury or illness deserves generous sympathy. One is tempted to laugh at the poor young lover who was hard at work in a car parked unobtrusively between hedgerows, and in his haste to satisfy natural desires had suffered a painful, but not too serious, injury: human flesh caught between the teeth of a hard metal zip. The ambulance crew has to keep its thoughts to itself until the patient has been safely treated and conveyed, if necessary, to further medical care.

Several years ago one of my colleagues at Greenford, Clive Swain, an ambulanceman with tact, understanding and a sense of humour, received a call one early shift to a most unusual case. A Perivale resident had dialled 999 in a state of some anxiety. He explained to Control that he had been attacked by a vacuum cleaner, or at least that is what it sounded like. Clive and Peter on Greenford 1 were sent to investigate.

A middle-aged man with receding hair nervously peered round the door when Clive rang the bell. His face was pale and his lips trembled. 'Ambulance?'

Opening the door wider, he stood awkwardly, clutching his dressing-gown just below his abdomen. 'Won't you come in.' Clive and Peter marched forward. Clive had already decided that the man was not having a heart attack, stroke or other sudden illness, but there was something odd about the whole situation. 'What's the problem?' he asked.

'Well,' gasped the patient, stepping backwards uncomfortably. 'I sort of had an accident with my vacuum cleaner.' Peter looked puzzled. 'I was doing some housework using the long attachment, and well, it happened.'

'What happened?' Clive wanted to know.

'Well, you see I was only wearing my dressing-gown, with nothing underneath, and the blessed thing sprung open, you see.'

'Yes?' Clive sounded doubtful; the story was sounding more and more ridiculous.

'Well the cleaning nozzle sort of grabbed me.' The man swallowed nervously between the last two words.

'Grabbed you?'

'Yes ... er ... here.' The patient pulled the dressing-gown apart to reveal his injury. Clive pulled away the tea-towel covering the man's private parts and immediately reached for a number 3 ambulance dressing. 'Nasty,' he remarked, as Peter too observed the extent of the wound. 'You may need a few stitches, gov'nor.'

'Yes, righto.' The gentleman looked relieved and pleased that there were no more questions. They took him to the Central Middlesex Hospital, and helped the man out of his embarrassment by discussing everything but his delicate injury. Clive was not naïve enough to believe the man's feeble story, but he diplomatically avoided the issue. At the accident unit, the patient was put in a cubicle while Clive cornered a sister to give her an outline of the case. The nurse smiled when she heard the story.

'What a naughty man!' she chuckled, walking towards the cubicle. As the curtains were drawn, Clive noticed that the man turned bright red. 'Oh, hello Mrs Cane,' he bleated unhappily. 'I never knew you worked here.'

'Mr Simpson! Yes, I've been here a few months now.'

'You know each other?' asked the ambulanceman, surprised.

'Very well. Mr Simpson is my next-door neighbour.'

Clive could not help smirking. 'That's nice.'

Contact with other emergency services—the Fire Brigade and Police—can have its humorous side. The police maintain friendly links with ambulance personnel and often pop in to our stations if they have a few moments to spare. Once a police traffic crew sat in the Greenford messroom, enjoying a cup of coffee. I asked why so many police vehicles had passed the ambulance station that morning. 'I'd rather not talk about it, Glen,' said one constable, looking a little uneasy. This, of course, only made me more curious, and I pressed for an explanation.

'Well, it wasn't really our fault; we feel sure it was all down to our radio controller at headquarters. Only he says that it wasn't his mistake, as he had the information in writing. You see, we were on patrol just off Hanger Lane when we got this message: "Stolen van proceeding along A40, load of guns aboard. Stop vehicle and arrest driver." Then they gave all the details. So we pursued the van after sighting it at Perivale Lane, and since we were chasing a haul of guns we called for assistance. I mean, it could easily have been a bunch of terrorists.'

'That's why there were so many police vehicles.'

'Yes. When we eventually stopped the van, we rushed the driver, who gave up without a struggle, searched him and waited for an armed unit to move in and surround the van before we opened up the back doors.'

'What did you find? A load of guns?'

'No, actually a load of buns.'

On another occasion a police crew was involved in a road accident. A traffic division car had crashed with another vehicle, and the police driver was white as an ambulance-woman treated him for shock. 'Are you all right?' she asked.

The constable nodded, and then his face suddenly became a healthier pink. 'Where's my mate?' he bellowed.

'He's fine,' said the attendant, trying to reassure him as she looked at the police patrol car and saloon taxi twisted together in the centre of the road.

'I don't care if he's broken both his legs. I want words with him, this is his fault! He definitely needs his bloody eyes and head examined.' The ambulancewoman tried to calm the officer down, and eventually she got the full story.

The police had been on a routine patrol. The officer, in the passenger seat, was busy trying out a new flavour of crisps while the driver helped himself periodically so that he could give a second opinion. The police car reached a junction where the driver was unable to see traffic coming from the left. He asked his colleague, 'Is there anything left?'

'No,' came the reply.

Then came the collision.

The complications and embarrassment of situation comedy on television, too, are often the result of arriving at 'the wrong end of the stick'. On my job I have quite often had to contend with such misunderstandings, only seeing the lighter side after the event. I worked with a lad of my own age several years ago, Alan Collins, a decent sort who was ready to do anything for someone in need. We became 'green' and available outside the accident centre at Northwick Park Hospital, Harrow, and I was about to reach for the radio to report our availability to Red Base, when a head poked through the sliding window next to me. It was a lady in her seventies, quaintly dressed with a light brown hat, matching overcoat, gloves and a veil.

'Excuse me,' she said timidly. 'I wonder if you could tell me if you're going anywhere near Harrow?'

We instantly recognised this as a request for a free ride, but neither Alan nor I had the heart to give a flat refusal. 'Well, love, the thing is, we're from Greenford Ambulance Station and that's in the opposite direction, I'm afraid.'

The old lady looked so sad. I looked at Alan to see if he was feeling the same as I was. 'Tell you what, dear, I'll radio through and see if we can go back via Harrow. But no promises.' She smiled, clutching her handbag.

'What are you going to say?' asked Alan.

'Oh, I shall just say that the nursing staff asked us to take a patient home after treatment. I'm sure they won't mind.' I guessed correctly and asked the gleeful lady to climb aboard. Alan took her name and address, and we drove down the ramp from the casualty department. We were quite pleased with ourselves; this was our good deed for the day. Alan pulled into the Harrow street the lady wanted and stopped outside the house. But she seemed anxious. 'Here we are,' I prompted her. 'It's home, sweet home.'

'Not here!' she exclaimed, shaking her head emphatically. 'I don't live here.'

'Yes, dear, this is the address you gave us!'

'Well it's not my house,' the lady said sharply. Asking Alan to keep an eye on her, I ran up to the door of number 11 and knocked several times but got no reply. A neighbour eventually called to me from her doorstep: 'The lady has already been taken.'

'You mean Mrs Pearson?'

'That's right. The doctor had a bit of a job getting her out. She's a little senile, you know. Another ambulance took her about an hour ago.'

'A short lady, in her seventies in a brown hat with a veil and gloves and coat?'

'That's her.'

I looked up to the skies, praying that the ground beneath would swallow me. 'Must be a mistake,' I chirped unconvincingly, and tripped as I turned around to make an escape to the ambulance. I could see that Alan was about to let the old lady out of the vehicle, and shouted to him frantically: 'No, no! It's OK!' I pulled his arm from the door handle. 'Get back to the hospital—quickly! I'll explain later.' Fortunately Alan did not ask questions and returned to the cab. I jumped into the rear of the ambulance and sat the lady down.

'Let me out!' she insisted. 'This *is* my house. Let me out this instant!' Getting back to casualty proved more difficult than the outward journey as the sweet old lady changed into a sour old crow. As we approached the accident unit, we could see several porters and security staff around, apparently searching the area. I put two and two together and got out of the vehicle to find the duty sister and make my peace. 'Sister, we've found a little old lady.' The nurse turned full circle at these words.

'Where is she?'

'In our ambulance—we—er—found her wandering about.'

'Thank God! We were just about to call the police.'

I hurried back to the ambulance, where Alan was helping Mrs Pearson. We handed her over to the nursing staff, and I then enlightened my mystified colleague. 'Never again, Alan, no more good deeds for little old ladies until we've checked them out.'

Ambulancemen certainly meet all kinds of people during their work—the happy, the sad, the good, the bad and the mad.

Last year a call came in: 'Call Red Accident. It's an RTA outside the parade of shops near Medway Drive, Perivale. Car on fire at 15.31 RW.'

The ambulance crew found a 1978 saloon car, its front section ablaze, and traffic and pedestrians lining the road to get a good look. The attendant rushed out with his satchel; his colleague reached for a fire extinguisher. As they approached the blazing car they saw a man who appeared to be changing the rear wheel! The attendant shouted to him to move back, but he took no notice. It then became clear what he was doing: unbelievably he was syphoning fuel from the petrol tank. The crew had to move him forcibly away from the car, as he shouted abuse at them, struggling.

'But petrol's so damn expensive—and I've only just filled up.'

Trying to deal with people who do not speak English can be difficult and it is, of course, a problem to assess the symptoms of such patients. Calls to Southall in west London often involve a crew in dealing with large Asian households without one person able to give the crew any help. Inevitably, out of all the confusion caused by language difficulties, some humour emerges.

Many years ago, in the days of canvas stretchers and metal poles, a crew went to Southall to attend an Indian who had been knocked over by a push-bike and had sustained various minor injuries. The crew decided to 'treat for the worst' and brought out a rigid stretcher. The Indian had suffered more than bruising; his turban, in its original shape, lay in the street.

The ambulancemen moved the patient on to the stretcher after a brief examination and assessment, made difficult because of the lack of communication. They reassured the shaken man as best they could—but forgot the cultural complications. Taking their positions at each end of the stretcher, they prepared to lift it, but the patient screamed out. They replaced it on the ground and again did their best to calm the man.

'Don't worry, you'll be OK. We want to help you,' they said, as soothingly as they could. The patient looked much calmer, and the crew tried again to lift the stretcher. 'Eeek!' screamed the casualty, and a further stream of Indian followed. 'Put him down, put him down,' commanded the attendant. 'You must keep calm' he said to the patient, patting his shoulder. 'We'll try again.' For the third time, as the crew began to lift, the unhappy patient gave a blood-curdling yell. By this time a large group of onlookers had gathered. A young man pushed through the crowd and spoke to the ambulance attendant. 'Excuse me,' he said politely. 'I speak the man's language. He says you are standing on his hair!'

To end this chapter, I would like to reproduce an article from the London Ambulance Service internal magazine *Londam*, by kind permission of the editor.

Why do you need an ambulance?

People tend to say some odd things when they dial 999, and Red Base Control have gathered, with quite kindly amusement, some of the odder replies from members of the public when asked 'Why do you require an ambulance?'

'My husband has lost half a bucket of blood from his brain, and it is all coming down his nose.'

'My wife is getting labour pains every three minutes and they are about eight grunts long.'

'My mate is injured, he's just driven his three-wheeler over an inspection pit.'

'My husband has terrible pains in his stomach. I think he needs one those stirrup-pump things.'

'My wife has just conceived!' (A very breathless male.)

'Can I send a telegram? Can I have a taxi? Oh, bloody hell, can I have an ambulance, my wife has started labour.'

'I have just had sexual intercourse for the first time and my legs feel all wobbly.' (Caller female. Advice given to caller. No further calls received.)

'My wife is bleeding from her regina.'

'I have just had a man on the floor and he is injured.' (Matron of an old people's home.)

'My husband has had a hysterectomy and it's gone wrong.' (Vasectomy?)

'My boyfriend has a bad cut on his head.' 'How did he do it?' 'He started getting sexually aroused and I hit him on the head with the Ewbank.'

8

Who Cares Wins

'Who Dares Wins' is the now familiar motto of the SAS paratroopers who stormed the Iranian Embassy siege last month. But for the LAS, an equally worthy group of emergency forces, a more appropriate motto might be 'Who Cares Wins'.
                    Ealing Gazette, Friday, 13 June 1980

That being an ambulanceman is more than just taking sick people to hospital must be clear enough to anyone reading this book. We are certainly not in the same league as the SAS but there are times when we face danger—a group of aggressive rioters perhaps, or an undetonated explosive device. One man who has had his fair share of risk is London's second in command, the Assistant Chief Ambulance Officer, John Moss MBE. Mr Moss joined the Service in 1948 and has dedicated his life to ambulance work. It was once said of him: 'If he were cut in half, like a stick of seaside rock, printed throughout his frame would be the words "Ambulance Service".'

Mr Moss is the first to acknowledge that the demands of his job and the manner in which he chooses to meet them rarely place him at the top of popularity polls. Nevertheless, on most major calls, many of which have a strong element of risk, he is there to advise and work alongside crews. 'I cannot expect ambulance personnel to do something that I am not prepared to do myself,' is his motto, and he means it. Apart from major incidents such as the Moorgate train disaster (looked at in the next chapter), he has organised Ambulance Service attendance at political incidents such as the Iranian Embassy siege, and at two similar sieges, Balcombe Street and the Spaghetti House, Knightsbridge.

The Storming of the Iranian Embassy

On 30 April 1980, at a terraced building in central London, twenty-five hostages were imprisoned by gunmen at the Iranian Embassy, Princes Gate. The siege lasted for six days, and ended in the dramatic armed military assault that was seen by millions of television viewers.

Throughout the siege, while politics were left to the politicians, security and safety to the police and, eventually, the rescue of hostages to the SAS, the care, treatment and transport of casualties were the responsibility of the Ambulance Service. No one knew when the hostages would be released, if at all, and so a constant vigil had to be maintained by the Service, a routine procedure at most sieges.

In the evening of day 1, the area around Princes Gate, Ennismore Gardens, Kensington Road and Exhibition Road was sealed off. No one in the vicinity of the Embassy moved except for armed 'special patrol group' police. The two ambulances on scene had to watch and wait, with back-up assistance available in the outskirts of the area.

On the second day a hostage, Chris Cramer of the BBC, was taken to St Stephens Hospital with possible dysentery. Iranian demonstrators massed at the Albert Hall side of the police cordon in Kensington Gore. Scuffles broke out and ambulance crews dealt with two patients with suspected fractures; one was a police officer, the other a student. Throughout the siege, Mr Moss was kept informed of police activity as far as possible. At some point the Service would be required to convey the hostages to medical aid, but no one could say when. Nevertheless, the major-incident trailer, which carried rigid stretchers, blankets and medical equipment, was ordered to move unobtrusively near to the besieged building.

The final day of the siege, 6 May, was the most dramatic. At 12.56 three shots were heard inside the building. Senior officials prepared to end the siege by force, and Mr Moss ordered seven ambulances to attend.

Ambulancemen Rick Taub and Jim Cambridge, a crew from Hillingdon, were in the W12 area at 15.40, having just

dealt with an overdose case. Jim, the attendant, called Red
Base from Hammersmith Hospital, reporting their availab-
ility. 'Think we might move you to the siege,' suggested the
Controller.

'Fine, we're more than willing.'

'Roger then, up to the Natural History Museum and stand
by.'

Rick and Jim, an advanced trained crew, had heard a lot
about the siege, both from the extensive television coverage
and from their own colleagues who were involved, and they
felt it was time they had a slice of the action.

At 18.35 the final phase of the siege began. Rick and Jim
were second in a line of eight vehicles (from a total of fourteen
ambulances at the scene). The police SPG was reported to be
on immediate standby, and twenty minutes later a 'patient'
was rolled from the Embassy steps, shot dead. Further
killings were threatened, one every half hour. Armed police
piled out of their coaches and took up their position in a show
of force. The chatter over police radios increased, and
ambulance crews stood ready.

At 19.23 the SAS assault began. An almighty explosion
rocked the ambulances, taking crews, police officers and other
related personnel entirely by surprise. A fusillade of shots and
screams filled the air. 'They've blown the bloody place up!'
exclaimed Jim, horrified. Two more explosions made the
ground tremble, while at least eight SAS men on the Embassy
roof began to abseil down ropes at the rear of the building,
and their colleagues made a frontal assault, armed with plastic
explosives and stun grenades. Tear gas was also used and
affected everybody. Rick felt the gas tighten his chest and
sting his eyes. Despite the coughing and spluttering, a senior
officer ordered ambulances to move forward so that they
would be as close as possible to the casualties. 'Right, lads,
let's make a move. I want the attendants to follow me up to the
Embassy, but for goodness sake keep your heads down.'
Bursts of automatic machine-gun fire could be heard as well
as single shots, as a line of ambulance personnel made its way
to the danger zone.

As Jim left the ambulance, Rick shouted after him. 'Make

sure you keep well out of sight, mate, I'm not ready to get a new partner yet!' A second team of four volunteer ambulance attendants, led by John Moss, also moved forward. The apprehensive unit had no idea what to expect—there had been reports that all the hostages had been shot. Mr Moss realised that it would be necessary to cross the front of the building. He crouched, signalling to his rescue party, and tried to attract the attention of the police cordon, whose guns pointed ominously in their direction. Halfway across the front of the building, a hooded gunman lurched into view and stopped the Assistant Chief and his group abruptly. Mr Moss peered down the barrel of a sub-machine gun. It was a tense moment: the un-military looking armed individual could have been a terrorist or a British soldier. Fortunately the officer used the magic word 'Ambulance' and the fearsome-looking marksman gestured the party to proceed.

On the other side of the Embassy, the large ambulance detachment had taken shelter among armed police in flak jackets. One officer turned to Jim: 'This is no place for you, mate; you lot don't get paid to be shot at.' The officer, realising the danger, commanded them to withdraw and reapproach the building. Mr Moss, on the other side, issued the following order: 'Seek, treat and remove.' Vehicles were relocated and the first group of casualties was met. Rick and Jim received the first and most seriously injured victim, brought out by armed police on a stretcher. They had no idea who this man was, but without speculating on his identity began to assess his condition. Amid sporadic bursts of gunfire, they found that their shaking patient had minor facial injuries and a wound in his leg where he had been shot. He was in a state of considerable anxiety, shouting and screaming about the possibility of being attacked again. Rick tried to calm him and found it necessary to get an armed police officer to stand guard on the ambulance steps to show their patient that he was being protected, so that the crew could set up an intravenous infusion for him. The man gradually became more coherent and calmer. He began to talk of his experience, offering his card to Rick. It read: 'Dr Gholam-Ali Afrouz, Chargé d'Affaires' (equivalent to Ambassador).

As other crews treated and conveyed their patients, the first inside details of the siege began to emerge. The hostages spoke of the immense horror they felt as terrorists—and in one case a fellow hostage—were killed before their eyes. One hostage had escaped death when an assassin's bullet was deflected off a 50p piece in his top shirt-pocket.

The 128-hour siege had involved sixty-seven ambulance crews and numerous senior officers over the six days. A total of twenty-nine people, five of whom were removed before the SAS assault took place, were attended to and conveyed by the Ambulance Service from the Iranian Embassy.

In his report on the siege, Mr Moss recorded the following:

> Throughout this protracted incident, crews and officers endured many hours of inactivity with patience and good humour, yet remained sufficiently alert to respond with alacrity when their services were required. All our staff on scene were exposed to varying degrees of personal danger but none was found wanting. I must stress the bravery shown by the four ambulancemen who crossed the field of fire armed only with medical kits—at a time when armed police were sensibly occupying sheltered positions in bullet-proof waistcoats.

Northern Ireland

A bitter phase to some, conjuring up images of insurrection, violence, civil warfare and innocent suffering. As an ambulanceman, I often think of my Belfast colleagues spending busy shifts attending to bomb-blast victims and the survivors of sniper fire. I imagine serious fires and daily explosions caused by uncontrolled terrorism in the streets of Londonderry and Armagh. Curiously, however, the most common call-out for the Belfast Ambulance Service is a road-traffic accident. Bombings and politically motivated incidents causing injury to others come quite low on the statistics tables. An ambulanceman serving in the Central Area of Northern Ireland, who lives and works in the Belfast district that covers calls to the well-publicised Falls Road, talked to me at length about his sometimes risky occupation. Alan Rogers (an alias for obvious reasons), a married man in his forties, has served for well over ten years in the Ambulance

Service. He is a dedicated man, committed entirely to the international principles of his profession, ignoring religious backgrounds, political divisions, colour and social class.

Northern Ireland has a population of approximately one and a half million. Belfast and its suburbs is the most densely populated region, East Belfast being the busiest place for calls. The Service has approximately 540 mobile staff and 260 vehicles, including a large accident and emergency ambulance for major incidents. In Belfast, fourteen front-line crews meet the daily work flow, but, unlike their London equivalents, they deal with all types of cases—non-urgent as well as 999 calls. This means a crew can be attending a serious accident at one moment and taking a geriatric case to a local hospital the next. The work is varied, and of 600 calls received in a twenty-four hour period, only about sixty would be 999 calls.

Alan's job is made easier by the local public's attitude to ambulances. Generally, if immediate assistance is required, crews are permitted to go freely into otherwise forbidden areas; ambulances are regarded as being above politics, neutral vehicles for the sick and injured. There are times when a self-styled soldier from a 'peace-keeping' force will insist on travelling with the ambulance crews during their duties in his territory or district. When a man with an automatic pistol offers his company it is an offer the crew does not refuse, even though they then become a possible target for the opposing side. Alan remembers having to plead with a rifle-holding gunman to go away, declining his 'kind offer of protection' and pointing out that he and his colleagues stood a high chance of being caught in any ensuing crossfire.

Although incidents concerning explosive devices are not commonplace, there have been times when the Ambulance Service's resources have been stretched to the limits by bombings. Pub explosions mean large numbers of dead or injured. Proper crowd control is impossible, and no one heeds the warnings of the police about further possible booby-trap detonations, as survivors search the rubble for friends and relatives.

In such circumstances Alan's work becomes a nightmare.

Not only is it impossible for him to treat first the person with the worst injuries—always his chief concern—but he is constantly aware of the dangers of the capriciousness of the people around him and of possible further bombs set to catch the unsuspecting officials.

After one bomb blast Alan treated a seriously injured victim under appalling conditions only to find when he had managed to get the patient back to where he had parked the ambulance that the vehicle was no longer there. Fearful and impatient people had used the ambulance to take their own less seriously injured friends to hospital. Alan and his partner were left to cope as best they could with a dying patient.

Self-reliance, heroism, valour and gallantry are best left aside in the streets of Northern Ireland: ambulancemen are as vulnerable as anyone else. Crimes of violence, reprisals and vigilante executions are among the horrifying call-outs. 'Knee-capping' for example is one of the commoner punishments for informers and those who have assaulted women or robbed for personal gain. After major terrorist incidents, ambulancemen may have no patients at all; only mortified and badly mutilated corpses remain.

Perhaps the saddest event that Alan remembers was the untimely death of a senior officer in the Central Ambulance Station at the Royal Victoria Hospital. Fireworks, rather like Chinese crackers, were heard going off in the station officer's room. When duty crews went to investigate, several gunmen emerged, guns aloft, and made good their exit, leaving behind the bullet-ridden body of Robin Shields and a handful of spent shells. He had been hit seven times in the head and chest as he sat at his desk. Despite all the trained ambulance personnel in the Station and the ready equipped vehicles outside, there was nothing that could be done. Mr Shields had served in the Ambulance Service for fourteen years; he was forty-four years old when he was murdered. The motive for the shooting is still not clear: the reasons given by his killers were disputed by authorities.

Alan Rogers has an unenviable job. Although his work is not all blood and political violence, the recurring crimes of violence would concern me deeply. I admire his resolution and pluck in accepting a job that frequently brings him in direct contact with appalling injuries while he and his colleagues are themselves in some danger.

Bombings: London

On 27 March 1976, with 15,000 people filling the vast interior of Olympia Hall, an explosive device was detonated on the first floor. The bomb, estimated as a two-pounder, had been planted in a plastic waste-bin close to a food stand around which a large crowd had gathered to watch a demonstration. Ideal Home Exhibitions are well attended, and the numbers of people at the Exhibition hindered the rescue operation.

Four ambulances were sent to Olympia, the first crew to arrive estimating that there would be at least twenty patients (in fact there were sixty, including an off-duty ambulance-woman, who despite her injuries reported to the Incident Officer to be enlisted as part of the rescue team). As with so many bombings, there was the possibility that a second device would go off, and at 17.14 hours, approximately half an hour after the explosion, the Police were told that there was a second bomb in the hall. As further ambulances moved in, the chances that crews, police and other helpers might be injured increased.

If another explosion had occurred, it would not have been the first time that emergency workers had been caught unawares. The bomb at the Tower of London on 17 July 1974 was perhaps a little more devastating. Although only one patient died, at least nineteen people, many of them children, were severely injured. A two-minute warning was given to a newspaper, hardly long enough to dial 999 before a device of at least 12lb exploded in the Mortar Room at the base of the White Tower. It was the height of the tourist season, and there were many visitors to the Tower that day.

It was ironic that the bomb exploded in a room in which weapons had lain unused for years only to be transformed by the explosion into deadly pieces of shrapnel, which shattered bones and tore flesh. The ambulance crews that were summoned saw several badly injured children, while less seriously injured youngsters and their families screamed uncontrollably in terror. Six or seven children, none of whom spoke much English, attempted to nurse their burned faces in the black, smoky atmosphere.

Meanwhile 15,000 other sightseers were swiftly evacuated, most of them needing little prompting, as the first group of seriously injured was treated and taken to St Bartholomew's Hospital, leaving the remaining ambulance teams, assisted by warders of the Tower of London, to deal with the other patients.

Since 1973, many explosive devices have been detonated in London and hundreds of people have been injured. Such call-outs always engender the strongest emotions in all concerned, yet like our colleagues in Northern Ireland, our primary concern as ambulancemen is for the patient. The whos and whys are not our business while we are on duty.

Bomb Incidents in London
Main call outs 1973–6
(ECV = Emergency Control Vehicle)

Date	Location	Vehicles sent	Casual-ties	Remarks
08.03.73	Great Scotland Yard, SW1	11	36	
08.03.73	Central Criminal Court	11+ECV	103	
10.09.73	King's Cross BR Station	4+ECV	5	
10.09.73	Euston BR Station	7+ECV	8	
12.09.73	Lower Sloane Street, SW1	2+ECV	2	
20.09.73	Duke of York Barracks, SW3	3+ECV	5	
17.12.73	Brompton Road, SW3	1	1	Letter bomb
18.12.73	Thorney Street, SW1	5+ECV	30	Explosion heard in Central Control
18.12.73	Horticultural Hall, SW1	4+ECV	6	Parcel bomb in temporary sorting office
18.12.73	Roman Way, N7	6+ECV	3	Nearby flats damaged; OAPs cared for by ambulancemen until emergency accommodation arranged

Date	Location	Vehicles sent	Casual-ties	Remarks
19.12.73	Heath Street, NW3	2＋ECV	0	Damage only
19.12.73	Sorting Office, W1	2＋ECV	1	Letter bomb
21.12.73	Leicester Square, W1	4＋ECV	2	Call from ambulance passing scene
22.12.73	National Liberal Club, SW1	2＋ECV	1	
22.12.73	Swiss Centre, W1	2＋ECV	0	One other bomb at scene defused
22.12.73	Shooters Hill Police Station	1	0	Letter bomb
23.12.73	Centre Point, WC1	1	0	Two explosions
24.12.73	Harrods, SW1	0	0	Bomb defused
24.12.73	Finchley Road, NW3	5＋ECV	6	
26.12.73	Victoria Street, SW1	2＋ECV	1	
19.05.74	Heathrow Airport, Car Park 1	2＋2 ECV	0	Three minor casualties treated at scene
17.06.74	House of Commons, SW1	5	9	
17.07.74	Tower of London	14＋ECV＋ 2 coaches	42	All but four casualties removed by LAS
22.10.74	Royal Overseas Club, SW1	4	3	
23.10.74	Harrow School	2	0	Unexploded bomb; ambulance stood by until explosion occurred
07.11.74	King's Arms P.H., SE18	6＋ECV	34	
25.11.74	Pentonville Road, NW1	3	2	
25.11.74	Piccadilly, SW1	4＋ECV	7	
25.11.74	Victoria Street, SW1	3＋ECV	1	
27.11.74	Tite Street, SW3	3＋ECV	9	Two explosions; casualties included 4 police and 2 ambulancemen
30.11.74	Little Chester Street, W1	3	5	Second unexploded bomb found nearby
17.12.74	Draycott Avenue, SW3	3	1	
17.12.74	Bloomsbury Tel. Exchange	2	3	
19.12.74	Oxford Street, W1	2	3	

Date	Location	Vehicles sent	Casual- ties	Remarks
21.12.74	Harrods, SW1	4+ECV	0	
23.01.75	Forest Road, E17	2+ECV	3	
27.01.75	Old Bond Street	1	1	
27.01.75	High Street, Kensington	3	3	
27.01.75	Victoria Street, SW1	2	2	
27.08.75	Caterham Arms P.H.	4	8	Assisting Surrey Ambulance Service
29.08.75	Kensington Church Street, W8	2	1	
05.09.75	Hilton Hotel, Park Lane	8	34	A further 22 casualties made own way to hospital
15.09.75	Callcott Street, W8	1	1	Letter bomb; casualty refused hospital treatment
15.09.75	Berkeley Square, W1	1	1	
22.09.75	Portman Hotel, W1	3+ECV	1	
28.09.75	Oxford Street, W1	3+ECV	2	
09.10.75	Green Park Tube, SW1	7	18	Ambulance passing scene at time
21.10.75	Whipps Cross Hospital	20	0	Bomb due to explode at midnight; hospital evacuated during search
23.10.75	Campden Hill Square, W8	2	2	Car bomb
29.10.75	Mount Street, W1	9	19	
03.11.75	Connaught Square, W1	4	2	Car bomb
12.11.75	Scott's Restaurant, W1	4	10	
18.11.75	Walton Street, SW3	9+ECV	17	
20.12.75	Biddy Mulligans P.H., NW6	4	5	
14.02.76	Brown Street, W1	3	2	
21.02.76	Selfridges, W1	4	5	Casualties included heart-attack case; unexploded bomb found nearby
21.02.76	Kendal Street, W2	2	0	Car bomb
01.03.76	Cromwell Road	2	1	
04.03.76	Cannon Street Station	7	8	Explosion on empty train

Date	Location	Vehicles sent	Casual-ties	Remarks
15.03.76	West Ham Tube	6	6	Bomb on train; driver shot dead by terrorist
16.03.76	Wood Green Tube	2	1	Explosion on empty train
27.03.76	Ideal Home Exhibition	15+ECV	84	

Riots

The Police, Ambulance Service and allied organisations are the only people present at riots who have not chosen to be there. Emergency workers have no axe to grind and would, if given a choice, prefer to be well clear of such events. Rioters, demonstrators and protestors give little thought to the crews caught up in conflicts: flying bricks do not distinguish among targets and are as likely to hit an ambulanceman as a demonstrator.

Southall, which is near to where I work, has been the scene of many rallies and protest marches, which culminated in the death of Blair Peach on 23 April 1979. Standing by for an imminent riot is like waiting to go over a World War I trench into enemy fire. Bottles, stones, bricks and any other missiles that come to hand are thrown, apparently at random, hitting the Police and fellow demonstrators alike. Police horses have paint, ball bearings and ammonia thrown at them. Disorder leads to chaos, and the chaos leads to many casualties.

One of the worst years for public marches and rallies was 1977. The Grunwick factory demonstration of 11 July produced thirty patients, and the final casualty toll after the Lewisham National Front March of 13 August was 103. Later on that same month, the Notting Hill Carnival brought 310 patients, all needing ambulance care and treatment before possible admission to a hospital casualty unit.

In July 1981, a wave of riots hit many British cities on a massive scale. During a large public disturbance in Southall a crew from my station became victims of a frenzied mob. The ambulance was responding to a police call for assistance, and was met by a hostile crowd that had already overturned and set fire to a police car. A brick was thrown at the windscreen, which shattered into pieces. The driver received a serious eye injury and slumped helplessly to one side, while his attendant faced the club-brandishing youths. Only his quick thinking foiled their attempts to enter the cab and further assault the crew—without hesitation, he pushed himself half-way onto the driving seat and accelerated away.

Subsequent riots up and down the country put great strain on ambulance personnel, as attacks during the performance of their duties became more frequent. Ambulance crews became the easier targets once the police donned protective helmets and took up riot shields.

Death of an Ambulanceman

The work of the Police Force and Fire Brigade occasionally claims the lives of officers. Police officers may be the victim of armed criminals, while firemen have always to be ready to face overpowering flames or collapsing walls and roofs. Few people would suspect that ambulancemen ever have to face such dangers, but on 1 September 1975, ambulanceman Terry N. Wilkinson became the third victim of a mad gunman. On the previous day Terry Wilkinson, a quiet, unassuming man, was asked by a colleague if he would swap shifts and take his night-shift in exchange for a day-shift. Terry agreed, and the following day came on duty at 22.00. About half an hour later, a car pulled up outside a semi-detached house in Lambourne Road, Leicester. The driver got out and, seeing his ex-wife chatting to some neighbours at the front gate, pulled out a double-barrelled shotgun and fired it at point-blank range, killing one of the neighbours. The man's ex-wife ran into the house with her ten-year-old son, and they barricaded themselves in an upstairs room. The murderer, Sabi Nickoloff, shattered a window with the butt of his gun and climbed into the house, carrying a can of petrol. What he was trying to achieve at this point is beyond comprehension, but his act had alerted Constable Acton who lived in an opposite house and who immediately called for police assistance. Constable Acton rushed out into the street to the shot neighbour but was startled by more windows being smashed and the sound of a further shot from inside the house. The screams of the mother and child could also be heard. Nickoloff then started a small fire on the staircase. With the assistance of another neighbour, Mr Back, Constable Acton managed to free the hostages. They placed a ladder against an upstairs window as far out of sight of Nickoloff as possible, and carried down first the boy and then the frightened woman.

Meanwhile, Constables Christian and Galloway had arrived, and when they learnt what Nickoloff had done, they decided to attempt a rear entry into the house. Before they could do so, two more shots rang out. Rushing to the front of the house, they found the body of a police sergeant lying shot in the road. He was still alive; a woman police constable with him was also wounded, but less seriously.

At 22.37 hours Leicester Ambulance Control received a 999 call from the Police: 'A shooting in Lambourne Road, Leicester.' A front-line vehicle, crewed by Terry Wilkinson and Gerald Oakley, was despatched at 22.38 and arrived four minutes later. Police officers put the crew in the picture, explaining the danger. Terry's first concern was the wounded police sergeant, who was still moving and had to be treated as soon as possible.

Ambulanceman Wilkinson decided that, since driving the ambulance to provide a shield was too dangerous, he and his colleague, together with the police, would push the vehicle into a position that would give shelter from the gunman. This would give only partial protection: to pull the injured policeman to safety, Terry knew that he was going to have to break cover and brave the danger from the front-bedroom window. Terry duly leaned forward to grasp the police sergeant, his colleague behind him ready to help. He never got the chance. A single shot killed the ambulanceman. Further shots slightly injured Constables Dickman and Proudman.

Gerald Oakley crawled to the offside ambulance door to summon further assistance on the ambulance radio since the injured police officers were unable to get to their own transmitters. Constable Christian, who attempted to radio from his panda car, was shot at and slightly injured. The police sheltered behind their vehicles and the stationary ambulance while the surviving ambulanceman made his move. A further shot shattered the ambulance windscreen, but Gerald pressed on and succeeded in pulling out the radio microphone, which fell on to the cab floor. He managed to call for assistance, his voice trembling as he gulped for air.

To protect those trapped near the ambulance, police reinforcements arranged for the street lighting to be extinguished. Two Fire Brigade vehicles were summoned so that they could shield police as they approached the house. However, all was soon over. As the first engine drew level with the house, the fire took hold and spread through the building. Nickoloff was seen clambering out on to the sill of a front upstairs window. His foot slipped, causing him to drop his weapon, which discharged both barrels as it hit the ground; then he too fell into the front garden, where after a fierce struggle he was overpowered and arrested.

After the incident several awards were issued to the police, ambulancemen and members of the public who had risked their lives. Gerald Oakley was awarded the Queen's Gallantry Medal; Terry Wilkinson received posthumously the Queen's Commendation for Brave Conduct.

Terry Wilkinson will never be forgotten by the nation's Ambulance Service as a man who committed a gallant act. True to the traditions of his profession, he displayed an unselfish concern for his patient, above and beyond the call of duty.

9

Stand By:
We have a Major Incident

On Friday morning, 28 February 1975, John Moss was on leave. It was a pleasant enough February morning, with the sun trying to shine, and the Senior Officer was all set to take full advantage of the day. His telephone rang at ten minutes past nine; it was the duty co-ordinator at Red Base. 'Sorry to disturb you, sir, but I thought you'd like to know that there is a four-ambulance attendance for an underground accident. A train has gone through the buffers.' The duty officer explained that the incident would probably be closed soon, and rang off, with further apologies for disturbing his superior.

Mr Moss resumed his late breakfast, only to be interrupted ten minutes later. The same officer had more details: 'Just to update you, sixteen casualties have now been moved, with a report of further patients trapped. I will keep you informed if there are any further developments.'

John Moss sat back uneasily in his chair. Something inside him was ringing an alarm bell. He dialled Central Control's number and asked for the duty co-ordinator. Mr Moss was aware that similar accidents were a fairly common event on London's underground; trains would often go through the buffers and there would be a handful of shocked patients. Yet this call did not seem to be in the same category: all the other cases were dealt with in half an hour, but now nearly an hour had elapsed. 'Moss again, where is this incident exactly?'

'Moorgate, sir.'

'Right, I'm going to attend.' At this stage, and in common with a great many other nearby emergency service men, Mr Moss was unaware of the gravity of the incident. He decided to make his way first to St Bartholomew's Hospital to assess the situation there.

The original call to Moorgate came at 08.48 from the direct line of the London Transport Executive. The request for an ambulance was brief—'train driver injured'—but since it was rush hour and the trains ran to full capacity, two ambulances were immediately despatched. A mobile Ambulance Superintendent was also despatched from Red Base to give a full report of the situation. The first vehicle arrived at 08.54, only six minutes after the first call. Ambulanceman Ronald Perkins, from Shoreditch Station, was an attendant that day, and it was his responsibility to make the first approach. Inside the building he could not immediately find a member of the station staff and even when he did so the man showed little knowledge of the call-out and went on selling tickets.

As he went down the stairs to the platforms Ron thought that the incident must be only trivial, but as he neared the platforms he could detect a strong smell of smoke. He went further down into the underground station but was still unchallenged and even occasionally jostled by a commuter. A little further down, he began to inhale airborne dirt particles and falling dust. At the bottom entrance to the platform, a man was propped against a wall. He appeared 'winded' and was in a state of shock. Then, from within the dim interior of the station platform came a group of passengers. At first Ron thought they were all coloured people; in fact they were passengers whose faces were covered with soot and grime.

Ron told his partner to deal with anyone who required treatment while he sent for help. He scrambled up the stairway and, assuming there had been a 'shunt' with multiple minor casualties, sent out a priority call for six more ambulances before racing back to the dark and gloomy platform. He made straight for the mouth of the tunnel where he could see a train standing motionless, some of its carriages inside the pitch-black opening at the end of platform 9. Only now did he realise the magnitude of the incident he was dealing with. It looked as if there had been a head-on collision of two trains, with one 'telescoping' into the other.

Walking casualties continued to emerge from the three nearest carriages, which were not too badly damaged. Some of the injured were clutching cut hands and nursing an assortment of minor wounds; others were simply shaken, milling around dazed. It was clear to Ron that they needed guidance and he instantly asked for two of the most capable and least badly injured passengers to take the lead and organise a human chain, with one patient holding the hand or arm of another. In this fashion, two groups of passengers helped each other to the safety of the upper levels of the station, well away from the danger area. Meanwhile, Ron dashed back to the ambulance radio, arriving outside the station breathless but at least in breathable air. He hastily called a further priority message, a phrase that only a handful of ambulance people have ever used: 'Shoreditch 1, make this a major emergency.' He gasped for breath: 'It's a serious train crash; Fire Brigade and Police to scene.'

At the station entrance Ron met a police officer on a motor cycle; the ambulanceman explained what had happened as briefly as possible, and, as two more emergency ambulances had by now arrived, he organised the crews, before dashing back fifty-seven feet beneath the London streets. The everyday scenes of commuters going to work and people wandering about the shops that Ron left at street level contrasted starkly with the horror on platform 9. Growing numbers of casualties continued to be treated on the platform, while those who were shaking off the numbing grip of shock began to voice their fears. There was no co-ordination of the rescue attempts until senior officers from the three emergency services arrived. Firemen, police and more ambulance crews converged in droves at the tube station and, after the initial surprise at the horror of the accident, set to work to free the living and sustain life.

Two distinct endeavours were now taking place at Moorgate. One team of rescuers began to try to free those unfortunate passengers who were trapped but, mercifully, still alive. Another group continued to treat and comfort those who were brought out of the wreckage. It was a unique disaster that would be known as the worst in the long history of London's underground system. Those passengers in the front carriages who were still alive cried, prayed and otherwise consoled themselves, as the realisation of what had happened grew. The trapped survivors had to listen to the last cries of many who had perished in the lonely darkness, sounds that would haunt them for ever. Panic and cold fear gripped the buried passengers. Some of them were trapped in steel cages, surrounded by jagged slivers of glass and the torn remains of the commuter train. The passengers included a woman police officer who was trapped by one foot. Together with a businessman she attempted to keep calm as the air in the carriage became foul and the temperature rose steadily. The bodies of fellow-passengers were constant reminders of the ghastly outcome of their fateful journey.

There was little time or opportunity for ambulance staff to stop and discuss anything else but how best to cope with the task in hand. There was exceptionally good communication among the emergency services. Major emergencies place an enormous emphasis on teamwork; co-operation, back-up and mutual assistance are essential if the rescue operation is to be executed with the minimum fuss and loss of life. No one service should assume total command or responsibility, nor should there be lack of organisation as one group of rescue workers awaits another.

At about 10.00 hours, a senior Red Base officer made his way to Moorgate to see the extent of the catastrophe for himself. Ambulances were parked outside the entrance to the underground station, and the sound of two-tone horns echoed everywhere. The choking stench, thick smoke and filth exuded from the station's lower depths became worse, but the ambulance and fire personnel engaged in the rescue could not be deterred. The escalator no longer functioned and only one naked bulb lit platform 9. The firemen searching the wreckage for survivors had to use hand-held torches. Victims who had not survived the head-on crash were seen by the rescuers but, sadly, they had to be ignored; the only priority was to release the living, and the dead were moved only if more room was required to work in.

The Officer observed the growing numbers of rescuers and felt that perhaps too many men were present in the confined space. He began to organise tasks for ambulance staff in the stifling discomfort. His duty was clearly to co-ordinate the treatment and removal of patients, maintaining constant liaison with Red Base Control and the medical team that had arrived from St Bartholomew's Hospital. He soon found it necessary to instruct exhausted ambulance staff to retire to rest, which they would do unwillingly and only under direct orders.

The main obstruction facing the rescuers was the twisted metal shell of the train, which repelled all attempts to breach it. Firemen worked relentlessly in teams, as ambulance crews treated those trapped people who could be reached and those who could be freed. Pain-relief gas was administered to many, and ambulancemen worked in the gloomy shadows to immobilise fractures. During the rescue operation the temperature reached 40°C (104°F); the heat inevitably produced a second wave of casualties as some of the fire fighters and ambulance workers collapsed with fatigue and lack of sufficiently oxygenated air. Salt tablets and capsules were issued to all, although there was an acute shortage of drinking water.

The only exit for passengers released from the front carriages was through a side window, which made the task even more difficult and delicate for ambulance teams. Experienced staff were supplemented by ambulance instructors and trainees straight from their classrooms. The trainees, who did not even possess uniforms, were used as stretcher-bearers, while experienced colleagues assessed and treated casualties.

Just after 10 o'clock a second medical team arrived from the London Hospital to support and assist the first medical unit already on scene. The London Ambulance Service's own medical officer, Dr Haigh, was closely involved in the emergency, offering advice and direct assistance to the uniformed rescuers.

The rescue procedures were arduous and painful for victims and rescuers alike. Extricating passengers took time, as no more than two or three firemen could work on the metal walls at any one time. By mid-morning twenty people had been released from a prison, but there were still many trapped further inside the tunnel. One girl died before she could be released, her back wedged and immovable against the roof that crushed her from above. It is not often that an ambulance crew has to stand and watch a person's life slip away without being able to raise a finger. Yet even with physicians and surgeons close at hand, nothing could be done. The reactions of survivors varied. Shock made patients hysterical, so that they either sobbed uncontrollably or laughed themselves to tears. Some casualties became rude and offensive because of their acute anxiety.

As time passed, the rescue became more organised. Generators were installed to purify the atmosphere within, while the Salvation Army and WRVS offered food and drink to the rescuers. News agencies were transmitting the sad details of the Moorgate disaster worldwide, and a large group of curious Londoners, kept at a distance by police, gathered outside the station's main entrance. Others, more helpful, offered blood at local hospitals, and many sympathetic taxi drivers offered free transport for this purpose.

It was a long time before the real nature of the crash was fully appreciated. The driver of a rush-hour train had failed to stop at Moorgate Station for reasons that are unknown even today. Instead of slowing down, the train gathered speed and crashed headlong into the solid concrete of a blind tunnel. Six carriages, as London Transport later found, had been 'concertina'd' together, the first three cars receiving the worst damage. The force of the crash caused the first carriage to jack-knife, its rear section being crammed roofwards as the second carriage forced a path underneath. The third carriage hurtled up and over the rear of the carriage ahead of it.

As the day's rescue attempts progressed, off-duty ambulance, police and fire personnel flooded to the scene, eager to help their colleagues. This happens at almost all major incidents and, although not expected, is always appreciated.

Well into the afternoon, only two live victims remained in the wrecked train. One was the woman police officer, Margaret Liles, the other was the businessman; they kept each other company as best they could. It was a struggle to release them, and as evening crept on, surgeons reluctantly decided that they would have to amputate the policewoman's foot. Under the most difficult conditions, these last two survivors were eventually taken by ambulancemen after twelve hours of painful confinement.

The rest of the operation, which took several days, involved the removal of the corpses. Protective clothing and face-masks had to be used as the risk of disease became a real concern. The final body was released only after four days of cutting through the crippled carriages.

On 5 March, at 09.45 hours, the Ambulance Service was finally dismissed. During the period of greatest activity at Moorgate, between 09.00 and 17.00 hours on 28 February, the London Ambulance Service had responded to 761 other emergencies in London. A total of 1,741 calls were dealt with during the twenty-four hours of 28 February.

The final official figures for the disaster stood at 41 dead, 76 injured. A total of 80 ambulance personnel, together with countless numbers of volunteer ambulance staff, had been committed to the one call. It was a combined effort with numerous other services that impressed people all over the world. It is comforting that such major incidents are rare; also that there are frequent 'mock-ups' so that the three emergency services keep their standard procedures well rehearsed.

I have been involved personally in only one major incident, and then only indirectly. It occurred in Ealing in 1973 and is known as the 'Ealing Train Crash'. Eight people were killed and 73 injured when two trains collided, upturning one carriage. This was the 17.18 Paddington to Oxford service, carrying 650 Christmas shoppers. Access to the train was possible only along a narrow alley between two houses, through a back garden and over a smashed fence to a ledge, from which rescuers had to descend to the tracks.

The other major emergency that sticks in my memory is the air disaster at Staines in 1972. This occurred by the Staines bypass near the Crooked Billet roundabout, at about 17.50 hours, which is a bad time of day for any emergency work through the rush-hour traffic. A BEA Trident plummeted to the ground after being airborne for only a matter of minutes.

The wreckage was devastating and the death toll horrifying. All the passengers in the shattered tail section were killed; one patient was removed when ambulance crews arrived but resuscitation attempts were not successful.

It is interesting to note that there was much initial confusion about this incident, rather like Moorgate. The first ambulances to be sent to the scene were unaware of what was waiting for them; one of them was called to a 'road traffic accident'.

Aircraft incidents, not necessarily leading to a disaster, are common at Heathrow Airport. The ambulance stations surrounding London Airport all have special 'yodel' alarms, and when these are activated by a direct line crews on station man their vehicles and go to designated points on the airport perimeter, further instructions being received over the air as they move. The 'turn out' of ambulances may be for an aircraft fire, an undercarriage failure or any mechanical defect that constitutes a potential hazard for an incoming aircraft.

Motorways are dangerous places at the best of times. I have often pulled over on the hard shoulder after seeing an accident on the opposite carriageway, only to find that it is impossible to cross the three lanes to reach it. An ambulance has always to be sent from a station that is on the 'right' side of the carriageway, and this is just as well for all concerned. The speed of some motorway traffic, sometimes over 100 miles an hour, could easily destroy patient, ambulance, crew and car-driver in a few seconds, leaving only a trail of motor parts and the remains of several human beings. The dangers are multiplied when a motorway is icy, foggy or snowbound. The same motorway madness persists, causing large-scale blood-shed in the vicious crashes that ensue. A 'pile-up' of thirty or forty cars is exactly that, and has devastating results for passengers. An ambulance crew working in such a situation is always alarmed at the prospect of a further accident while dealing with injured patients, some of who may be trapped. The police make every effort to control and organise traffic flows, but they are not always first on the scene.

Whatever the major emergency, the Ambulance Service, together with the other services, must remain on constant standby, ready to act at a moment's notice. As a direct result of experience in large-scale incidents, all three emergency services and hospital medical teams are becoming better organised, better equipped and more effectively managed. If nothing else, the unfortunate victims of past major accidents will indirectly help those who, unfortunately, find themselves in similar situations in the future.

Putting it into Perspective

The media may be responsible for the general public's misconceptions of the Ambulance Service. Television in particular sometimes paints misleading pictures of ambulance duties, rarely presenting a true-to-life impression.

I recollect watching an episode of 'The Sweeney'. In the middle of an action-packed shoot-out, the villain was 'blasted' at close range and required urgent medical treatment. After the well-used 'Call for an ambulance!' phrase was sung out, followed by the two-tone horns, along came a somewhat outdated ambulance, which screeched to a halt, its headlights blazing. As the rear doors swung open, two ambulancemen in black and white uniforms hopped out with a stretcher, closely followed by a nurse in a grey smock. The St John Ambulance Brigade had arrived! Not that I have anything against this fine organisation, but its members would be the first to point out that they do not answer 999 calls in London.

A television unit descended upon a Central London ambulance station on one occasion to film a sequence with an ambulance and crew for a television play. The director asked the crew to 'scoop up' its patient, heave him into the back of the vehicle and depart at breakneck speed, with both driver and attendant sitting in the front. Needless to say the crew, and indeed the entire station, refused to co-operate, explaining that it never happened like this in real life and that a bad impression would be given of ambulance personnel. The director was not convinced but left after realising that he could not have his own way, and the film unit was temporarily forced to abandon its script.

I only hope this book has helped to put ambulance work

into some sort of perspective. The role of the ambulance person is rapidly changing. In the last ten years improvements in equipment and training have been revolutionary, compared with those of the previous twenty years. Nevertheless there is still a long way to go.

I have already mentioned paramedic and advanced training. In London there is a scheme to train selected personnel in the techniques of intubation and infusion, both forms of emergency treatment usually only practised by doctors and some specially trained nurses. They are life-saving measures that have already proved their worth in the hands of ambulance crews. 'Endotracheal intubation' is the insertion of a long airtube into the lungs in order to maintain a clear airway in an unconscious patient, or an unobstructed route for resuscitation measures. Intravenous infusion—infusing certain fluids directly into a patient's vein—is an important life-sustaining treatment, especially in cases of severe blood loss.

My advanced training programme was intensive, with lectures, demonstrations, frequent tests and written exams. There was also a practical period spent in operating theatres under the wing of a consultant anaesthetist. I was most fortunate in being attached to St James' Hospital, Balham, with a most skilled consultant, who made every effort to train me to a high standard, and I spent three weeks putting my theoretical knowledge into practice with her enthusiastic guidance. Since qualifying (and it is the consultant who has the final say in the matter), I have used my skills quite frequently. On one or two occasions, without the specialised treatment, my patient would undoubtedly have died.

On 16 November 1979 my colleague Jim Lock and I received a call to a Tesco supermarket on the Greenford Road. It was given as a 'collapse' and we responded to the case at 09.55 hours. Approaching the scene I could see a woman lying on the pavement. Beside her was a young woman whose pale face showed her anxiety. From the ambulance cab I was able to diagnose a possible cardiac arrest; the patient looked blue and there was no sign of life. I learned that the woman had only just stopped breathing, seconds before our arrival.

The informed bystander was a State Registered Nurse.

We got to work immediately, ventilating the woman's lungs with a 'bag and mask' unit. I could tell the airway needed suction, and this was carried out with our portable aspirator. After clearing the throat and entrance to the lungs, I decided to intubate the patient with Jim's assistance. The nurse was eager to help although she was related to, and therefore emotionally involved with, the patient, and I asked her to commence cardiac massage. Gradually the patient took on a more healthy colour, and by the time we arrived at Ealing Hospital I could detect a faint pulse. We had a chance.

I must say, however, that trying to resuscitate a patient in the back of a moving vehicle is an extremely difficult and hazardous operation. Many is the time I've nearly lost my teeth when using a plastic air introducer (Brook's airway) on a cardiac arrest, and trying to keep balance when the ambulance reels around corners is a tricky business. I have known crew members to be flung headlong into the driver's cab before now. So much depends on road conditions, other road-users and a partner who drives considerately.

I am pleased to say that our patient was eventually transferred to the intensive-care ward and discharged after ten days of therapy—100 per cent fit and healthy. A doctor assured us that her success was directly attributed to the advanced care we were able to provide at the scene.

Even so, some physicians and nurses are not in favour of ambulance staff receiving advanced training, although they never seem to offer a clear-cut reason why. Thankfully the majority of doctors are in full agreement with the principle of paramedic crews and it is hoped that such teams will be recognised officially, as they are in the United States, where top ambulance paramedics are trained in minor surgery.

In England the three ideal places to collapse, particularly if you are a heart patient, are Belfast, Bristol and Brighton. Each of these areas runs a cardiac ambulance scheme, and Bristol and Brighton have vehicles manned entirely by highly trained ambulance staff. I once had occasion to speak to Brighton's Chief Ambulance Officer, Mr Grainger, and was impressed by what he told me about the high success rate of heart-attack victims who are resuscitated by advanced crews.

Before 1971, when Brighton started its cardiac ambulance scheme, at least 50 per cent of all coronary patients attended to by crews died in the first hour of their attack, many on the way to hospital—a situation that has been drastically improved in the last decade. Through the painstaking care and enthusiasm of a consultant cardiologist, Dr Douglas Chamberlain, MD, FRCP, and his colleagues, the pioneers of the project, coronary patients were being saved on a large scale.

An unfortunate aspect of this breakthrough in ambulance technology is that the Brighton scheme is largely financed by public funds. Life, it seems, has a price after all and the Government is unable to supply anything but a small research grant. In London, advanced training is not officially recognised or encouraged, on the absurd grounds that hospitals are near and plentiful in the capital. Yet it only takes three minutes for a cardiac-arrest victim to die if untreated. Without advanced emergency care, their chances of survival may be low, even if they live next door to an accident and emergency unit.

Although Britain still has one of the best Ambulance Services in the world, there are places, such as the United States, Canada and Scandinavia, that would put us to shame. Other nations are following their lead, and Britain is in danger of being left behind in yet another field. It is up to the Dr Chamberlains to forge ahead and improve standards and training.

Perhaps those in power will see the need for improvements. Financial backing aimed specifically at increasing skills and equipment would go a long way. There will always be accidents and serious illnesses, and ambulance personnel will always be required. We cannot be replaced by machines or micro-chips. Our function remains the same: the critical care of accident and emergency patients. The more resources that are put into maintaining standards and training specialised personnel in the ambulance field, the better the investment for future generations. It would indeed be fascinating to look fifty years into the future. To have a 'state-registered ambulance technician' would give every potential accident victim a better chance of full recovery.

At the time of writing, the future of the Ambulance Service of this country is a little uncertain. There is a general trend to improve medical skills, and organisations such as the Association of Emergency Medical Technicians have this view in mind. However, I am sure greater progress would be made if the public were more aware of the need for better training so that they could support the ambulanceman's fight.

I have tried to explain the unique nature of ambulance work. There are few jobs left that offer as much varying interest, few careers that place such emphasis on the decision-making ability of the individual. I am sometimes surprised when I look back upon the time I have been an ambulanceman. I initially joined for twelve months before taking up a possible place in medical school; I have remained for eight years. Many of my colleagues also find themselves reluctant to change their job. It is not just the security but more a feeling of daily accomplishment through one's own personal endeavours, affecting other people's lives on occasions, by skilled and speedy action.

Having no set environment to work in also generates a great deal of interest through one's working day. I remember one shift during which I visited an embassy, a glue factory, Marks & Spencers and a prison, all within five hours. Only a job such as ambulance work would take someone inside such a variety of places in so short a space of time.

All these factors make ambulance duties appealing. Few people these days can honestly say that after several years in their employment they still actually look forward to going to work. Ambulance staff are perhaps some of the lucky few.

And so, in a few hours' time, I am again on call. I have no idea what I shall be called to do, who I shall meet or where I will travel in my eight-hour tour of duty. Whether I remain an ambulanceman for the rest of my working days, or for some reason leave the profession, I shall always acknowledge my Ambulance Service experience as having a deep and lasting effect on my thinking as an individual, giving me a profound appreciation of health and, most precious of all, life itself.

Appendix 1

Calling an Ambulance

Anyone may call for an ambulance, whether at home or in a public place. In the United Kingdom the service is free, apart from calls to road-traffic accidents, when a small charge is made, which can usually be reimbursed by the motor insurance company.

All telephones in Britain bear the well-known emergency instructions: 'Fire, Police, Ambulance: Dial 999.' These three digits connect the caller in the first instance to the telephone operator. After requesting one of the Services he is then put in direct contact with the relevant emergency control centre.

If an ambulance is required, the operator will connect the caller to a local or regional headquarters, operated by uniformed ambulance control officers. Most of these ambulance personnel have actually had first-hand experience of accident and emergency work; many are knowledgeable ambulance workers who have had many years 'on the road'. This is an important point to bear in mind when speaking with ambulance controllers, because they are well qualified to give first-aid advice to the flustered caller.

In London, the extensive control network of Red Base is situated at London Ambulance Headquarters, Waterloo Road, SE1. All calls originating in the Greater London area are passed to this vast centre that co-ordinates the work of every emergency ambulance in the nation's capital. By a powerful radio link, calls may be passed to mobile accident ambulances on the air as well as to ambulance stations. It is possible for an emergency vehicle as far north as St Albans to communicate with another in the depths of Surrey.

Problems that arise when ambulance assistance is summoned usually result from the caller being panic-stricken. Many is the occasion when all the control officer will hear is 'Send an ambulance, quick!', followed by the abrupt sound of a receiver being replaced. On other occasions, the calling party is rude or abusive, taking out the strain of the moment on the officer accepting the details.

An ambulance will normally be sent whenever a patient needs urgent hospital treatment. However, in cases where the individual requiring attention has a long-term illness (and is not dramatically worse), the caller is sometimes asked to refer to his own general practitioner. Many people believe it is their right to call an ambulance even if it is merely to be used as a taxi. This may, technically, be true, but surely not at the expense of depriving someone in far worse condition of a fully equipped emergency ambulance. While an ambulance is conveying Mr A to hospital (a resident in Wembley for example) with mild stomach pains, his neighbour Mrs B may suffer an acute heart attack. She will have to wait much longer for an emergency vehicle to come all the way from Park Royal or Greenford. Her nearest ambulance, and there is only one covering the Wembley area, is tied up with that thoughtless man who could have easily gone by taxi.

The opposite situation may also prevail. Some people are afraid of wasting ambulance time and try to make do, with fatal results. I remember seeing a car hurtle into the grounds of Central Middlesex Hospital, screeching to a halt outside the casualty entrance. On the back seat was a man, slumped backwards, his face deathly pale. He had been stabbed several times, and his rescuer had almost finished him off by not calling for ambulance assistance at the scene of the assault.

The rule to follow, therefore, is to telephone your own doctor in the first instance for non-urgent medical treatment. He or she may well arrange for an ambulance as a result. If a doctor cannot be reached, dial 999 and ask the control officer's advice. He too may feel that an ambulance is required. If he is in any doubt, he will send one regardless.

Always request an ambulance for any sudden illness such as chest pains, heart attacks, strokes, collapses and accidents in the home that need specialist treatment.

To summarise:
1   If you require an ambulance, or think you do but are not sure, dial 999 and seek advice.
2   When put through to the Ambulance Control, give the telephone number from where you are speaking and all relevant information. Speak slowly and clearly.
3   If possible, make sure that someone is manning the telephone from where you make your call, as the responding crew may require more information.
4   Look out for the ambulance approaching. It is a great help for the caller or someone on scene to flag the emergency vehicle down rather than let the crew hunt for house-numbers. While waiting for the ambulance it would be useful to jot down any details known about the patient: name, address, date of birth, history, next of kin, tablets being taken if any, etc.
5   Give all the necessary details to the crew when they arrive. They must be fully aware of all the facts. Based on information received and their assessment of the patient's condition, the ambulance attendant will begin the required emergency treatment.

Calling a Doctor

Everyone who subscribes to the National Health Service in Britain should be registered at a general practitioner's surgery. If this is not done, problems occur when a doctor is needed. People who move house often forget to change their physician and have a great deal of trouble when a medical crisis occurs. Not all doctors answer their own house-calls on a twenty-four-hour basis. Like everyone else, GPs need time to themselves, and as a result arrange for a locum doctor to take their place. This usually happens in the evenings after surgery and throughout the night; it means that patients can have medical attention at any time of the day or night, but not always from their own GP.

To call a family doctor, ring the surgery or emergency number given. If the surgery is closed, there will usually be a recorded message giving another telephone number, or the operator will provide an alternative number to dial. If there are problems in doing this and if the patient's condition is rapidly deteriorating, *telephone 999 (ambulance) and ask for advice.*

Going to the Casualty Department

Many people needing urgent treatment but who are capable of getting to the hospital under their own steam, do so. Here they will be treated for any accident, recent injury or sudden illness such as chest pain. A letter from a general practitioner is not necessary, although he or she will be informed of any subsequent medical treatment.

In the same way that emergency ambulances are often misused by the public, so too are local accident/emergency departments. Patients come in for treatment for their constipation, haemorrhoids, ingrowing toenails and acne.

In one north London Hospital that I regularly use in the course of my work, there is a large sign stating the following:

Your Accident and Emergency Department will treat:
Road traffic accidents; heart attacks; suicide attempts; fractures and dislocations; strokes; accidental self-poisoning; eye injuries; burns and scalds; acute abdominal conditions; new injuries; serious chest infections.

Your Accident and Emergency Department will not normally treat:
Athlete's foot; chronic backache; coughs and colds; conjunctivitis; constipation; corns and warts; diarrhoea; ear trouble and wax in ears; hayfever; headaches; ingrowing toenails; injuries more than 2 days old; rashes; sebaceous cysts; sore throats; social problems; toothache (see your dentist); urinary symptoms. See your General Practitioner.

Appendix 2
What can I do for a Patient until the Ambulance Arrives?

People often ask me 'What can I do while waiting for an ambulance?' The answer is not simple, for it obviously depends on what is wrong with the patient, and this is not always easy to discern if you have no medical training. Nevertheless, assuming that you do not possess a first-aid certificate—a useful qualification that anyone may obtain—but would like some guidelines on the subject, I will briefly summarise the main points.

A (Airway)   B (Breathing)   C (Circulation)

If you understand these three factors and have used this knowledge in relation to your patient, go no further. This is really all you need to know if an ambulance is on the way. The golden rule is not to move the casualty unless he is in further danger from burning or drowning, for example, as an ambulance crew will have all the experience and training to ensure the patient's condition is not made worse by being mishandled.

However, do ensure that your ABC has been carried out on the patient.

A (Airway)
Is the casualty's airway clear? If the patient is making funny gurgling sounds, or his face is going unusual shades of purple and blue, it is likely that his airway is obstructed. So clear it!
1 Remove false teeth if any. (Use your handkerchief if you are squeamish.)
2 Tilt the head back a little and ensure that the patient's tongue is not causing inadequate air intake.
3 Use your finger (bound by your handkerchief) and remove anything that threatens to choke the patient, eg vomit. If the patient is conscious he or she will be coughing and spluttering and doing the job themselves (see 'Choking').

If you have been successful so far, continue now to:

B (Breathing)
Is the patient breathing correctly? Is he breathing at all? How can you assess this for yourself? Well, try:
1. Placing your hand over their mouth and nose. Can you feel their warm breath? (Wet your hand if necessary.)
2 If you carry a mirror, put this up to the patient's open mouth. If the casualty is breathing, the mirror will mist up.
3 Look for chest movements. Can you see the chest rise and fall?
So, is the patient breathing?

If yes, then support the head so that the patient does not choke. (Do not lie him flat on his back!) If the patient is already on his side or front—good, provided that the head is facing down and to one side and that the airway is clear. Put your hand near to the mouth and nose periodically to 'feel' the breath and assure yourself that all is well.

If no, then you've got your work cut out! Ideally, you need someone who knows how to perform what is technically known as CPR (cardio-pulmonary resuscitation) and sometimes, poetically, as the 'Kiss of Life'. I am not going to go into this in any detail, as diagrams and a great deal of information would be required. However the basic principle is to: *(a)* clear the airway; *(b)* tilt the head back, pinching the nose and opening the mouth; and *(c)* breath deeply into the patient, watching for chest movement.

I strongly advise you to look this procedure up in any first-aid textbook, it could indeed prove life-saving. So many victims of heart attacks and electrocution are left by ignorant by-standers who have no idea what to do. Many of these patients could well have survived if treated immediately by CPR.

One small point: when performing this technique place *a cloth handkerchief, or other piece of material over the patient's mouth.* It will ensure that you are not put off too much by this drastic measure (unless you are male and are working on a nineteen-year-old blonde girl!), but if the patient vomits, I need not spell out the awful consequences. You will need an ambulance too!

C (Circulation)

Is the blood going round? An odd question you may think, but essential for life itself. If the patient stops breathing, it is almost certain that the heart will stop as well. If the heart no longer functions and there is no circulation, the brain will die in three minutes from lack of oxygen carried in the blood. CPR can prevent this, and again I refer you to a first-aid text book, to the section on cardiac massage. This action, performed on the chest of a patient without a pulse and who is not breathing, helps to circulate a percentage of the blood supply around the body.

The second point about circulation is if there is a break in it. That is to say, is the patient bleeding? Severe bleeding will also cause death. So prevent further bleeding:

1   By direct pressure. Use a clean cloth or something similar. (Infection is of secondary importance when the bleeding is very severe.) Then apply solid pressure.

2   *DO NOT* tie tourniquets. The use of tourniquets is dangerous, especially for the layman. On some occasions their use has led to the amputation of a patient's limb, a measure that could have been avoided if the tourniquet was not used. Tourniquets are

for the highly trained and not for 'green' first-aiders, especially if an ambulance has been called.

3   If possible, elevate the limb. If a patient is bleeding from the wrist, say, apply direct pressure and then raise the hand into the air, providing there are no fractures. (Blood has more difficulty going up hill.)

A B C: Important Points

1   Do not attempt CPR if your patient is breathing. (People do!)
2   *Stop* if you are successful. By continuing on a live patient you are likely to reverse your good work.
3   Take precautions when practising mouth-to-mouth resuscitation. If you are put off in any way, your patient has little or no chance.
4   Never do anything to a patient you are not sure about. If in doubt, don't! (But do use your commonsense.)

Other Injuries or Illnesses

Burns and Scalds

The main actions here are: *(a)* reduce heat; and *(b)* cut off the air supply to the affected area.

By immersing the affected limb in, for example, water you will be doing both the above. For other parts of the body apply clean, wet, preferably sterile, material or dressings. Continue to 'top up' the absorbent covering with cold, but not ice-cold, water.

In the Ambulance Service we carry clean plastic bags. These are filled with water and burned hands are placed inside. The bag is then sealed about the patient's wrist and he is taken to hospital with this 'goldfish bowl' arrangement (and much relief).

Two important points however:

1   Don't use forceful running water, as in the jet of a tap. This may further damage burned skin, causing pain. Always immerse into a container of still water (or, if water is not available, a harmless solution such as beer, milk or orange juice).
2   In cases of very severe and extensive burns, where the damage is extremely deep, only exclude air with clean material. The patient's nerve endings will have been destroyed and the casualty will not be in the sort of pain that warrants cold-water treatment.

Chest Pains

These are always something that should be checked, particularly in the over-35s. Do consult your doctor, or if the pain is severe call an ambulance immediately. While waiting for the crew, place the patient where there is plenty of air, near an open window, for instance. Reassure him and prevent agitation. Loosen tight clothing and keep him sitting up.

Childbirth

Let nature take its course. If you have decided to help with the delivery while waiting for the ambulance crew, do the following:

1   Wash your hands, scrubbing them thoroughly.
2   Calm the mother and check for signs of the baby emerging. A show of blood and the breaking of water about the baby's body usually occur first of all. Tell the mother not to bear down until the baby's head is clearly visible. (Not during contractions.)
3   As baby emerges, place one hand on the head and support it with the other.

Make sure the new born infant comes into the world *slowly*. (Be careful, babies are slippery.) Wrap baby warmly. *Do not cut* the cord. Finally, don't forget to congratulate the mother!

The other further action that should be taken is if: *(a)* the cord is around the baby's neck, in which case, ease it over the head gently; and *(b)* a membrane is covering the face—it should be torn away.

Choking

A person whose food goes down the 'wrong way' is seriously at risk of choking to death. Every year hundreds of people throughout Britain die this way. So what do you do in a crisis?

1   A child may be turned upside down, and if necessary thumped between the shoulder blades. Use your fingers to extract any foreign object. Use the *Heimlich Manoeuvre* (described below) if necessary.
2   An *adult* should also ideally be turned upside down, but this is difficult and requires several rescuers, so a recent technique, the *Heimlich Manoeuvre*, may be used, which has proved quite successful. *(a)* Go behind the casualty and link your arms in front of him. *(b)* Making a clenched-fist grip with both hands, apply the hold to the victim's upper abdomen (solar plexus). *(c)* With sudden sharp movements, pull back, until the object becomes dislodged in the mouth. *(d)* Remove the obstruction.

This technique is operated on the same principle as that of a cork flying out of a champagne bottle: the build-up of pressure in the bottle forces the cork (the obstruction) to fly out. The same thing happens when force is applied to the abdomen.

Diabetics

Assuming they complain of diabetic symptoms—ie weakness, headache, irritable, clammy skin, rapid pulse, and are known diabetics—simply give plenty of sugar, provided that they are conscious and alert. Perhaps sugar dissolved in water or milk; chocolate and biscuits can also be given. No harm is done if they are suffering from too much sugar in their bloodstream.

However, *do not* give anything to the semi-conscious or unconscious patient.

Electrocution
Turn off power supply, then consider your A B C. If the patient is all right, consider treating burns if any. Reassure.

Epilepsy
Most sufferers from epilepsy recover after an attack and decline medical aid. However if you have warning (usually from the patient himself) that an attack is imminent, put the patient in a place where he will not harm himself (on the floor, in a house). Steady his head and support it from harm. If possible, slip some material, like a folded handkerchief, between his teeth (but not if his teeth are already firmly clenched; nor should you risk your own fingers between his jaws—you may lose them altogether!). Apply gentle restraint during the seizure and maintain an adequate breathing posture.

Fractures
Do nothing. This is definitely a task for the arriving ambulance crew.

Glue stickers/sniffers
Two modern aspects for first-aid consideration.
1   Those stuck by powerful bonding agents, whether by accident or on purpose, should consider the use of nail-varnish remover. (Obviously a lady rescuer would be more successful here.)
2   Those overcome by glue sniffing should be observed for side-effects, and their airway maintained if they are rendered unconscious or succumbing to vomiting.

Heart Attacks
Reassure the patient and treat as for chest pains. Patients on tablets such as TNT should be helped to take the recommended dose under their tongue. Consider A B C if the patient becomes unconscious.

Infantile Convulsions
These are quite common in children, particularly if they have an infection causing a high temperature. Also, babies that are made too warm may have a fit. Undress the infant and, if you have a fan, use it. A tepid flannel on the forehead and back of the neck is also useful. (Reassure the mother.)

Overdose cases/poisonings
Reassure the patient but take no further steps while awaiting the ambulance. The tablets or substance in question should be kept for the arriving crew to inspect.

Strokes
If the patient is unconscious, revert to A B C; otherwise talk to him. Offer reassurance, even if you receive little acknowledgement that he is able to understand you.

Unconsciousness
Again, A B C is the rule. Keep a constant watch as the next stage is respiratory/cardiac arrest should the patient deteriorate.

Other Points

Drinks to patients   Avoid this practice, the patient may need an anaesthetic.

Taking observations   A pulse reading is useful to the ambulance crew, but far from essential. Leave the technical aspects to them; you should concentrate on making your patient feel better by following these guide lines and offering plenty of reassurance.

Medical diplomacy   Don't discuss the patient's condition where he or she can hear you. Don't fuss too much. It is essential the casualty does not become unduly concerned.

Be useful   Help the ambulance crew and work under its instructions when it arrives. After you have given all the details, step out of the way. The crew will surely call on you if it needs your assistance.

Lastly, please remember that all this information is merely an outline. Study a book on first aid.

Appendix 3

Equipment Carried on Emergency Ambulances

Attendant's satchel containing:

Front section: Brook airway; Guedel airway, large; Guedel airway, medium; Guedel airway, small; KY lubricating jelly; cervical collars (1 adult, 1 child).

Middle section: Roehampton burns dressing; dressings No 1; dressings No 2; dressings No 3; triangular bandages; roller bandages 3 inch; adhesive plasters; safety pins (card).

Rear section: insulated gloves; disposable gloves.

Driver's satchel containing:

Front section: Brook airway; Guedel airway, large; Guedel airway, medium; Guedel airway, small; KY lubricating jelly; cervical collars (1 adult, 1 child); Roehampton burns dressing.

Middle section: dressings No 1; dressings No 2; dressings No 3; safety pins (card).

Rear section: triangular bandages; roller bandages 3 inch; cotton wool, 1oz; adhesive plasters; adhesive plasters, 1 inch; disposable gloves; Resusci-bag; Resusci-bag, adult; Resusci-mask, child.

Venti masks; aspirator; flowmeter (and oxygen apparatus); entonox with mouthpiece; maternity pack; maternity blanket, small; maternity blanket, large; burns sheets.

Dressings case containing:

triangular bandages; roller bandages, 3 inch; cotton wool (1oz); dressings No 1; dressings No 2; dressings No 3; scissors on cord; safety pins, (cards of), roll of plaster, adhesive zinc oxide, 1 inch; assorted adhesive dressings.

Stretcher trolleys (with straps); stretcher poles; spreader bars; stretcher canvas; Furley stretcher; pillows; blankets; carrying chair; carrying sheet; hot-water bottles and covers; bedpan with cover; urine bottle; bowl, kidney; bowl, round with lid; vomit bags; drinking-water flask; disposable beakers; splints, wooden; Neil Robertson stretcher; splints, inflatable, half-arm; splints, inflatable, half-leg; splint, spinal with straps; orthopaedic stretcher with straps; manifold harness; deodorant spray; incontinence pads; feeding cup/eye bath; drip-bottle holder; spade terminal leads; rescue equipment; crowbar; retaining bars for anchorage (centre); waterproof sheets; hand-lamps; safety helmets; safety goggles; white coats; polythene bags, large, disposable; fluorescent jackets; map book; message pad; major emergency plan; clipboard; extension lead for Francis lamp; Francis lamp; fire extinguisher; inventory card; estate keys; IV drip stands; automatic resuscitator; radio transmitter.

Rescue equipment kept in sealed canvas bag:
Eclipse saw; crowbar, small; guideline, 12 yards; pliers (8 inch sidecutting); screwdriver, slot-head; screwdriver, Phillips-head; pipegrip or stilson; rescue knife (tied by lanyard to canvas bag).

Advanced crews also carry:
laryngoscope; Endotracheal tubes; Spencer Wells clamps; syringe; Magills forceps; stethoscope; blood-pressure apparatus; administration sets; various IV fluids; cannulae; miscellaneous equipment to supplement the above.

Appendix 4

Training Programme for Ambulance Students

Section 1:
1 The ambulance service within the National Health Service
2 Conditions of service for ambulance staff
3 Code of conduct
4 Hygiene and physical fitness
5 Duties of ambulance crews
6 Operational control
7 Radio procedure and communications
8 Long-distance journeys
9 Accident and sudden illness (emergency journeys)
10 Operation information and procedures (other patients)

Section 2:
1 Organs of the body
2 Skeletal system
3 Circulatory system
4 Respiratory system
5 Digestive system
6 Nervous system

Section 3:
1 Wounds and their treatment
2 Effects of injury; control of bleeding
3 Traumatic shock
4 Injuries to tendons, ligaments, joints and bones
5 Injuries to pelvis and spine
6 Care and management of head injuries
7 Care and management of maxillo facial injuries
8 Care and management of the unconscious patient
9 Chest injuries
10 Asphyxia and injuries to the respiratory system
11 Artificial ventilation
12 Cardiac compression
13 Use of suction equipment
14 Use of oral pharyngeal airway
15 Oxygen therapy
16 Use of entonox
17 Inflatable splints
18 Immobilisation and support
19 Burns and scalds
20 Poisoning
21 Effects of heat and cold
22 Ambulance patient report form

Section 4:
1 Lifting and handling of patients (various methods)
2 Lifting and handling of patients (use of carrying chair)
3 Lifting and handling of patients (use of sheet and pole)
4 Lifting and handling of patients (use of orthopaedic stretcher)
5 Lifting and handling of patients (use of Neil Robertson and Paraguard stretchers)
6 Knots and lashings
7 Patient positioning
8 Light rescue

Section 5:
1 The law and the ambulanceman
2 Co-operation with the Police and Fire Service
3 Major accidents
4 Dangerous loads
5 Motorway procedure

Section 6:
1 Mental illness and drug dependence
2 Management of violent patients
3 Artificial kidney patients
4 Infectious diseases (general)
5 Infectious diseases (smallpox)
6 Maternity
7 Premature babies; care and use of incubator
8 Infants and children

Section 7 (selected crews):
1 Advanced theory: cardiopulmonary systems, nervous system, lymphatic system
2 Advanced emergency-care techniques
3 Interpretation of vital signs, including blood pressure
4 Vene-puncture, intravenous infusion
5 Laryngoscopy, endotracheal intubation
6 Management of home dialysis patients
7 Advanced theory: cardiac illnesses
8 Operating theatre etiquette

Section 8 (some areas of Britain):
1 ECG interpretation
2 Drug administration (including atropine, lignocaine, dextramethasone)
3 Defibrillation procedure
4 Control of diabetics with glucogon (if indicated)
5 Use of oesophageal airway
6 Paediatric intubation
7 Venous cut down
8 Chest drainage

Appendix 5

Example of an Ambulance Test Paper

This example is included to show the standard required to pass a preliminary stage of advanced training for experienced personnel. (This is in fact a test paper I myself had to complete.)

Mid-Course Assessment
Time Limit 1½ Hours

1 (a) State three reasons why we intubate.
   (b) Describe step by step the procedure for endotracheal intubation.
   (c) What level of consciousness must this patient be in before intubation?
   (d) How do you know if you have passed the tube too far and intubated the right bronchus?
2 (a) What is the treatment of a patient with a flail segment of the left hand side of the chest?
   (b) What is a tension pneumothorax?
3 (a) What is emphysema?
   (b) Describe how it affects the lungs.
   (c) What does a patient suffering from emphysema look like and why?
4 (a) What is an aneurysm?
   (b) Describe how it affects the lungs.
   (c) What is myo-cardial infarction?
5   Describe step by step the procedure for setting up an intravenous infusion, including cannulation.
6 (a) What is the function of the vaso-motor centre?
   (b) Describe BP drop.
7 (a) What is dead space and how many ml?
   (b) What is the average residual air in a fit person?
   (c) What is meant by the term tidal volume?
   (d) When would you consider using the Heimlich Manoeuvre?
8 (a) When taking the blood pressure, what are you looking for in the readings you are taking?
   (b) What is meant by the rule of 100?
9   You are given an emergency call, a patient who is suffering from left ventricular failure. Describe what signs and symptoms you would expect to find and what treatment you would give.
10   If a patient is knocked out, regains consciousness, then goes out again, what could be wrong with him, if he is suffering from a head injury, and why?

Appendix 6

Common Questions and Answers

1 Where do ambulances come from?

On the whole in England, ambulances originate from accident or main ambulance stations, many of which may be near to a hospital. However the Ambulance Service is totally separate from hospitals where organisation and running are concerned. Hospital staff have no official jurisdiction over crews, who are responsible to their own superior officers.

2 Do all ambulances have blue lights and two-tones?

No, some vehicles are used only for out-patient work and are rarely used for anything of a more serious nature.

3 When are the blue lights and sirens used?

At the discretion of the crew, usually going to an emergency call (90 per cent of the time). Occasionally with a patient on board, depending on the circumstances.

4 Can the lights and sirens be used to avoid traffic hold-ups when proceeding on routine matters?

No.

5 Do you need a special licence to drive an ambulance?

No, a full licence is acceptable, but preferably 'clean'.

6 At what age can you join?

In London it is 21, though some candidates are accepted at 18. A few Services run a cadet scheme with a starting age of 16.

7 What are the hours?

Usually 40 hours a week on a shift rota (7 am to 3 pm; 3 pm to 11 pm; 11 pm to 7 am). Day work (8 am to 4 pm; 9 am to 5 pm; 10 am to 6 pm) is restricted to out-patient journeys.

8 Can an ambulance legally proceed through red traffic lights?

Yes, on an emergency, provided that the driver treats them as a 'give way' sign, proceeding with caution. An ambulance may also use the bus lanes and may park anywhere while on official business. Ambulances may exceed the speed limit when safe to do so, again if on an emergency.

9 What is the training like?

Quite intensive. An initial 2-week induction course leads the candidate into 6 weeks in the classroom. As with nurses, a period in front of the blackboard is supplemented by practical training and experience. There are plenty of written and oral exams. Trainees also go on a two-week police-style advanced driving course and a short spell in hospital to work alongside medical staff (ward rounds, casualty, operating theatres and delivery suites, etc).

After one year's experience, a trainee becomes qualified after much assessment. After several years of service, ambulance personnel, in certain Services, may apply to take advanced paramedical courses. (In London a written entrance exam is a prerequisite.)

10   Who keeps the ambulances clean?

The crews themselves. They are solely responsible for the state of their vehicle and the tidiness of the ambulance station.

11   If I call for an ambulance, may I choose the hospital to go to?

No, generally. Crews are instructed to take their patients to the nearest casualty receiving unit in the immediate area, unless otherwise arranged by a doctor.

12   What do crews do if called out during a meal?

Go hungry! Eating on duty is a risk—many is the delicious meal I've had to let go to waste. It's part of the job, unfortunately.

Appendix 7

The London Ambulance Service's Story

In February 1915 a new accident ambulance service was formed in London under the control of the Chief Officer of the Fire Brigade. During that year ambulance stations were opened at Fulham, Bloomsbury, Shoreditch, Newington, Lee and Brixton. Nine ambulances were provided, manned by an operative staff of fifty. Until this time, Londoners involved in accident or sudden illness in public places would have been moved by hand or wheeled litter, although the Metropolitan Asylums Board did provide an ambulance service to convey fever patients.

From the 2,405 calls recorded in 1915, the number increased over the years until, in 1928, 41,189 were received. Today, the figure for Greater London has risen to 420,000. To cope with the ever-increasing work, more ambulance stations were opened, and by 1929 the Service had 14 stations in commission, with 20 ambulances and a total staff of 165.

On 1 April 1930 the London County Council took over the ambulance services previously provided by the Metropolitan Asylums Board and 25 Boards of Guardians, including 6 large ambulance stations, 107 vehicles and a staff of 270. At the same time the Accident Section was transferred from the Fire Brigade to the Public Health Department.

At the outbreak of war in 1939, the LCC area had: 6 large ambulance stations; 16 accident ambulance stations; 200 vehicles (including ambulance-buses); 422 operative staff including superintendents and station officers. The London Ambulance Service formed the nucleus of the London Auxiliary Ambulance Service, which was created to deal with air-raid casualties. At its peak, the wartime service in Greater London included several thousand vehicles with over 10,000 auxiliary personnel. More than 100 additional stations were opened, some of them—and their personnel—suffering from enemy action. In London alone, 48,709 war casualties were removed to hospital and first-aid posts.

On 5 July 1948, the National Health Service Act placed on all local health authorities the duty to provide ambulance services free of charge. In fact in London the great majority of patients needing ambulance transport were already receiving it without charge. In 1965, with the creation of the Greater London Council, the nine existing services operating within its area were amalgamated into a single unit, and the London Ambulance Service thus became the largest of its kind in the world. Finally, from 1 April 1974 the Service became part of the reorganised National Health Service.

Acknowledgements

My gratitude to my friends and Service colleagues who rallied to support me in this project, with a special mention to Kathy Nye and the London Ambulance Service training school.

Index